Dana-Farber Cancer Institute Handbook Se

Lung Cancer

Edited by

Paul Lorigan
Senior Lecturer in Medical Oncology
Christie Hospital NHS Trust
Manchester, UK

Series Editor

Arthur T. Skarin
Associate Professor of Medicine
Harvard Medical School
Senior Attending Physician
Medical Director, Lowe Center for Thoracic Oncology
Dana-Farber Cancer Institute
Department of Medicine, Brigham and Women's Hospital
Boston, MA, USA

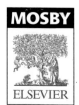

EDINBURGH LONDON NEW YORK OXFORD
PHILADELPHIA ST LOUIS SYDNEY TORONTO 2007

ELSEVIER
MOSBY

ISBN: 978 0 7234 3437 5

British Library Cataloguing in Publication Data
A catalogue record for this book is available from the British Library.

Library of Congress Cataloging in Publication Data
A catalog record for this book is available from the Library of Congress.

Note
Knowledge and best practice in this field are constantly changing. As new research and experience broaden our knowledge, changes in practice, treatment and drug therapy may become necessary or appropriate. Readers are advised to check the most current information provided (i) on procedures featured or (ii) by the manufacturer of each product to be administered, to verify the recommended dose or formula, the method and duration of administration, and contraindications. It is the responsibility of the practitioner, relying on their own experience and knowledge of the patient, to make diagnoses, to determine dosages and the best treatment for each individual patient, and to take all appropriate safety precautions. To the fullest extent of the law, neither the Publisher nor the Editors/Authors assume any liability for any injury and/or damage to persons or property arising out or related to any use of the material contained in this book.

The Publisher

Printed in China

Contents

Preface

The last 6 years have witnessed a dramatic change in our approach to, and expectations for, patients with lung cancer, across all histological subtypes and stages of disease. These changes have been driven by the outcomes of a number of well-designed randomized trials, supplemented by data from meta-analyses. The role of computed tomography (CT) screening in high-risk patients has been rigorously studied. The results of a large, non-randomized study (I-ELCAP) are very encouraging, and the outcome of a large US randomized study (National Lung Cancer Screening Trial) will be available at the end of the decade. Adjuvant therapy for patients with completely resected tumours has been convincingly shown to improve survival, and interest is now focussed on which stages to target and which drugs to use. Adjuvant radiotherapy for node-positive disease is to be revisited. Concurrent chemoradiotherapy is now accepted as standard of care for fit patients with locally advanced, inoperable disease; the role of surgery in patients downstaged by chemoradiotherapy is less clear.

Patients with advanced disease can expect to have improved survival and better symptom control with modern chemotherapy doublets than with older triplet regimens. Newer, targeted therapies, including growth factor receptor blockers and anti-angiogenic strategies, have resulted in significantly improved outcomes in particular patient groups, and have increased the opportunities for second- and third-line therapies.

For patients with small cell lung cancer, the optimum treatment regimens have been clearly defined, and the importance of radiotherapy timing, dose and fractionation are better understood. New randomized data on prophylactic cranial irradiation in limited and extensive stage disease will soon be available.

However, despite all of the above improvements, the majority of patients with lung cancer still die of their disease, and further improvements are needed across all areas.

This handbook combines a large collection of images and illustrations with a comprehensive review of all recent developments, referenced using key papers. It sets out to provide a detailed overview of the state of the art, with a clear indication of where new developments are likely to come from. We have opened the door on targeted therapy, are knocking on the door of CT screening, but still on the driveway when it comes to predictive biomarkers and personalized therapy.

Paul Lorigan
Senior Lecturer in Medical Oncology, Christie Hospital NHS Trust,
Manchester, UK

Contributors

Ramon Blanco, MD FACP
Chief of Pathology at Falmouth Hospital
Medical Director of Laboratories,
Cape Cod Healthcare and Martha's Vineyard Hospital
Falmouth, MA, USA

Joseph P. Eder, MD
Assistant Professor of Medicine, Harvard Medical School
Phase I Group
Medical Oncology Division
Dana-Farber Cancer Institute
Department of Medicine
Brigham and Women's Hospital
Boston, MA, USA

Christopher S. Lathan, MD MS MPH
Center for Outcomes and Policy Research
Lowe Center for Thoracic Oncology
Dana-Farber Cancer Institute
Boston, MA, USA

Janina A. Longtine, MD
Assistant Professor of Pathology, Harvard Medical School
Clinical Director, Molecular Biology Laboratory
Department of Pathology
Brigham and Women's Hospital
Boston, MA, USA

Ravi Salgia, MD PhD
Associate Professor of Medicine
Director, Thoracic Oncology Research Program
University of Chicago Hospitals
Chicago, IL, USA

Tad Wieczorek, MD
Instructor in Pathology, Harvard Medical School
Department of Pathology
Brigham and Women's Hospital
Boston, MA, USA

Acknowledgements

The work of the associate editors of the *Atlas of Diagnostic Oncology* needs to be acknowledged. Dr Maxine Jochelson (currently Director of Oncologic Radiology and Women's Imaging, Cedars-Sinai Medical Center, Los Angeles, CA) and Dr Robert Penny (currently Director of Hematopathology, Community and St Vincent's Hospital of Indianapolis, IN) assisted with the first edition. Their immense help in organizing and evaluating the radiographic and pathology material for the chapters contributed significantly to the success of the *Atlas*. The work of the associate editors of the third edition, Dr Kitt Shaffer, currently Cambridge City Hospital, Cambridge, MA and Dr Tad Wieczorek, Instructor in Pathology at Brigham and Women's Hospital, is also deeply appreciated. Their expertise was invaluable in emphasizing the illustrative and teaching aspects of the third edition. Without their hard work on the *Atlas of Diagnostic Oncology* this Handbook would not have been possible.

Acknowledgement also has to go to the editorial staff at Elsevier Ltd for their assistance in preparing the *Dana-Farber Cancer Institute Handbook Series*.

Introduction

Arthur T. Skarin

The *Dana-Farber Cancer Institute atlas of diagnostic oncology* was originally published in 1991 as a comprehensive reference and teaching aid in the various clinical, laboratory, pathological and radiological features of specific cancers. Because of the recent progress in understanding the molecular biology of cancer and the development of multiple novel chemotherapeutic agents it became apparent that there was a need for a combination of the teaching aspects of the *Atlas* with a review of modern therapeutic programmes available to cancer patients accompanied by recommendations. Thus arose the new *Dana-Farber Cancer Institute handbooks* of four common cancers – breast, colorectal, lung and prostate. Relevant sections of the 3rd edition of the *Atlas* have been updated and are now combined with new material, which includes treatment strategies.

The likelihood of developing cancer during one's lifetime is one in two for males and one in three for females, based on the 1998–2000 Surveillance, Epidemiology, and End Results database.[1] The median age at cancer diagnosis is 68 years for men and 65 years for women. The overall 5-year relative survival rate for all patients is 62.7% with considerable variation by cancer site and stage at diagnosis. The variation in cancer statistics over recent years in the US is depicted in Figures 1.1 and 1.2. The American Cancer Society estimated that in 2006 the total number of new cases would be 1,399,790 with 564,830 deaths (see Figure 1.3).[2] The death rate from all cancers combined has decreased by 1.5% per year since 1993 among men and by 0.8% per year since 1992 for women. The mortality rate in men has also continued to decrease for the three most common sites (lung/bronchus, colon/rectum and prostate) as well as for breast, and colon and rectum cancers in women. However, lung cancer deaths among women continue to increase slightly, paralleling the rise in cigarette smoking among women. Of interest, since 1999, cancer has surpassed heart disease as the leading cause of death for those under age 85 years; the reverse exists for those over age 85 years.[2]

Worldwide, an estimated 11 million new cases and 7 million cancer deaths occurred in 2002 while nearly 25 million people were living with

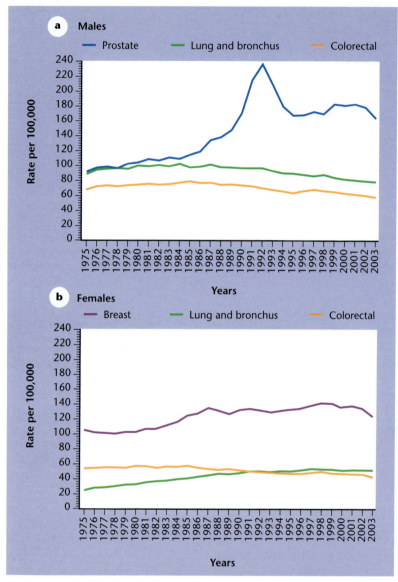

Fig. 1.1 Annual age-adjusted cancer incidence rates among (**a**) males and (**b**) females for selected cancers in the US, 1975–2003. Data from: Surveillance, Epidemiology, and End Results (SEER) program (http://seer.cancer.gov) SEER*Stat Database: Incidence – SEER 9 Regs Public-Use, Nov 2005 Sub (1973–2003), National Cancer Institute, DCCPS, Surveillance Research Program, Cancer Statistics Branch, released April 2006, based on the November 2005 submission.

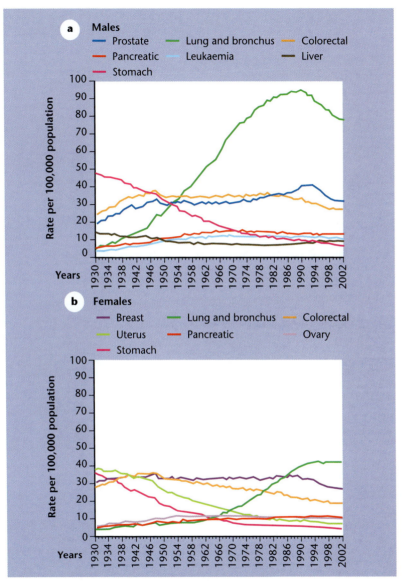

Fig. 1.2 Age-adjusted cancer death rates for selected cancers in the US between 1930 and 2002 for (**a**) males and (**b**) females. Source: US Mortality Public Use Data Tapes, 1960–2002, US Mortality Volumes, 1930–1959, National Center for Health Statistics, Centers for Disease Control and Prevention, 2005. Reproduced with permission from American Cancer Society. Cancer Facts and Figures 2006. Atlanta, American Cancer Society, Inc.

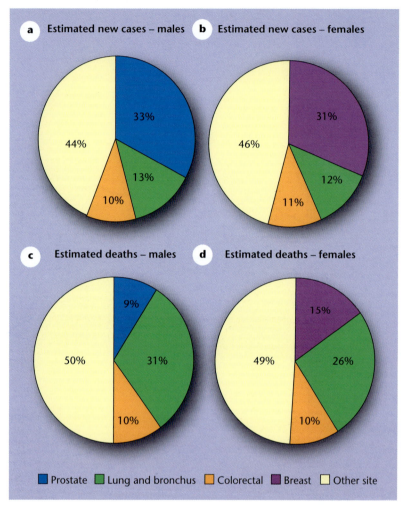

Fig. 1.3 Leading sites of new cancer cases and deaths – 2006 estimates. (a) Estimated new cases – males. (b) Estimated new cases – females. (c) Estimated deaths – males. (d) Estimated deaths – females. Source: American Cancer Society, Inc., Surveillance Research. Estimates of new cases are based on incidence rates from 1979 to 2002, National Cancer Institute's Surveillance, Epidemiology, and End Results program, nine oldest registries. Estimates of deaths are based on data from US Mortality Public Use Data Tapes, 1969–2003, National Center for Health Statistics, Centers for Disease Control and Prevention, 2006.

cancer.[3] Global disparities in cancer incidence, mortality and prevalence relate to genetic susceptibility and ageing, but also to modifiable risk factors such as tobacco use, infectious agents, diet (low fruit and vegetable consumption) and physical activity. Other modifiable factors include overweight/obesity, urban air pollution, indoor smoke from household fires, unsafe sex, and contaminated injections in healthcare settings.[4] At least one-third of world cancer deaths are felt to be preventable. The associations of established causes of human cancers have been categorized as chemicals and naturally occurring compounds, medicines and hormones, infectious agents and mixtures.[5] Lung cancer, for example, is the most common cancer in the world and the leading cause of cancer related mortality, with about 1,179,000 deaths per year. In order to counter the tobacco epidemic, the World Health Organization Framework Convention on Tobacco Control, organized in 2003, has proposed restrictions on advertising, established clean indoor air controls and strengthened legislation against tobacco smuggling.[6]

As a result of the improvements in healthcare and other factors, there is an increasing ageing population in the US and many other countries in the world. It has been estimated that the proportion of people over age 65 years will increase in the US from 12.6% in 2000 to 14.7% in 2015, and 20% in 2030.[7] This compares with 18.1% in Italy (used as a comparison as the oldest country in the world) in 2000, 22.2% in 2015, and 28.1% in 2030. Since the incidence of cancer increases with age, a rising number of cancer cases and deaths is predicted. Screening for cancer is therefore extremely important for early detection and subsequent cure. The annual screening recommendations by the American Cancer Society have been published.[8] Unfortunately, for lung cancer, there are no specific studies or tests, but rather thorough discussion by high-risk individuals (mainly cigarette smokers, those with emphysema, and especially those with a previous lung cancer) with their physician is recommended. While studies using low-dose spiral computed tomography scans show a higher percentage of low-stage resectable lung cancers than chest radiographs, decrease in mortality has as yet not been demonstrated.[9] An ongoing Prostate, Lung, Colon, and Ovary (PLCO) study addresses the question of whether screening asymptomatic persons for lung cancer is beneficial.[10] Several more years will be required before end results could dictate policy decisions.

Cancer prevention is extremely important and the progress in information technology has been recently reviewed.[11] Chemoprevention studies have been carried out for several cancers and also recently reviewed.[12] For lung cancer, unfortunately several randomized studies

Table 1.1 Molecular biomarkers associated with neoplasia characteristics[14]

Evading apoptosis

BCL-2, BAX, caspases, FAS, TNF receptor, DR5, IGF/PI3K/AKT, mTOR, p53, PTEN, *ras*, IL-3, NF-κB

Insensitivity to antigrowth signals

SMADs, pRb, cyclin-dependent kinases, MYC

Limitless replicative potential

hTERT, pRb, p53

Self-sufficiency in cell growth

Epidermal growth factor, platelet-derived growth factor, MAPK, PI3K

Sustained angiogenesis

VEGF, basic fibroblast growth factor, $\alpha_v\beta_3$, thrombospondin-1, hypoxia-inducible factor-1α

Tissue invasion and metastasis

Matrix metalloproteinases, MAPK, E-cadherin

BAX, BCL-2 associated X protein
BCL-2, B cell lymphoma 2
DR5, death receptor 5
FAS, fatty acid synthase
hTERT, human telomerase reverse transcriptase
IGF, insulin-like growth factor
IL, interleukin
MAPK, mitogen-activated protein kinase
mTOR, mammalian target of rapamycin
NF, nuclear factor
PI3K, phosphatidylinositol 3-kinase
pRb, retinoblastoma protein
PTEN, phosphatase and tensin homologue deleted on chromosome 10
TNF, tumour necrosis factor
VEGF, vascular endothelial growth factor

using alpha-tocopheral beta-carotene (ATBC), beta-carotene and retinol (CARET) and beta-carotene and aspirin (Physician's Health Study) as well as other studies have been negative.[12] Present studies include celecoxib in current and former smokers (with a surrogate endpoint of reversal of bronchial abnormal histology), an intergroup adjuvant study (E5597) using daily 200 µg selenium, and other trials using similar biomarkers and Ki-67 levels. Some recent studies are evaluating the role of novel targeted agents, active in advanced non-small cell lung cancer, in high-risk individuals in the chemoprevention setting. Progress in chemoprevention drug development is rapid and has been recently reviewed in detail.[13] The goals are to integrate the specific molecular biomarker expressions into the development of new agents for the chemoprevention of early intraepithelial neoplasia. The molecular targets summarized in this American Association for Cancer Research Task Force Report include anti-inflammatory/antioxidant agents, epigenetic modulation areas and signal transduction modulation targets. Six characteristics of neoplasms and the associated molecular targets that maybe adversely affected by chemoprevention or definitive treatment programmes are noted in Table 1.1.[14]

With completion of the Human Genome Project new knowledge has become available about genetic variations that can aid understanding the family history as a risk factor for most cancer types. Identification of mutations in genes may identify individuals at high risk for certain cancers (*BRCA1*, *BRCA2*, *p53*, *PTEN* and others); allowing for early detection, as well as increased understanding of the aetiological subtypes of cancer and inherited alterations in drug metabolism. This exciting field of molecular epidemiology may thus impact favourably on cancer prognosis.[15] The importance of the above underscores the need for collection and storage of adequate tissue for study.

The new information explosion in molecular biology has led to important discoveries in unique patterns of gene expression characteristic of certain malignancies.[16] This genetic expression profiling will not only be important for accurate diagnosis but for determining prognosis and candidates for certain therapies.[17]

Another new blossoming area of research is cancer proteomics.[18] In this field, as the result of carcinogenesis, abnormalities in protein networks extend outside the cancer cell to the tissue microenvironment in which exchange of cytokines, enzymes and other proteins occurs to the advantages of the malignant cell. These molecules can be identified and become the target for new diagnostic and/or therapeutic targets. Major progress is occurring in the proteomics field in the discovery of biomarkers that may be useful in predicting the clinical response to anticancer therapy.[19]

Major research advances have not only occurred during the past few years in cancer biology, genetics prevention and screening, but also in cancer treatment.[20] New standards of care for breast, lung and colon and other cancers became established during 2005. There is also evidence of an increasing number of newer targeted therapies that can improve survival in some of the most common cancers but are also active against several other malignancies. This applies to adjuvant chemotherapy after surgery as well as advanced disease (see Chapter 4). Targeted therapy has the advantage of oral administration for many agents, as well as directed attack on cancer cells, sparing most healthy cells including the hair and bone marrow. Of note, a detailed review of new and future therapeutic targets has been recently published.[21] Also, multidisciplinary treatment guidelines from the National Comprehensive Cancer Network for lung cancer have been recently updated.[22]

In each of our *Handbooks*, the authors review important aspects of each cancer, including epidemiology, diagnostic work-up and staging evaluation, with photographic examples of pathology subtypes and clinical presentations, all followed by an up-to-date detailed discussion of multimodality treatment programmes with current recommendations where necessary. In this book on lung cancer, Dr Christopher Lathan, attending physician on the Thoracic Service at Dana-Farber Cancer Institute, will review various aspects of comprehensive treatment including the use of new drugs and targeted agents. The importance of patient symptom management and quality of life efforts are also addressed.

REFERENCES

1. Gloeckler LA, Reichman ME, Riedel Lewis D, et al: Cancer survival and incidence from the Surveillance, Epidemiology, and End Results (SEER) program. Oncologist 2003; 8: 541–552.
2. Jemal A, Siegel R, Ward E, et al: Cancer statistics, 2006. CA Cancer J Clin 2006; 56: 106–130.
3. Kamangar F, Dores GM, Anderson WF: Patterns of cancer incidence, mortality, and prevalence across five continents: Defining priorities to reduce cancer disparities in different geographic regions of the world. J Clin Oncol 2006; 24(14); 2137–2150.
4. Ezzati M, Henley SJ, Lopez AD, Thun MJ: Role of smoking in global and regional cancer epidemiology: Current patterns and data needs. Int J Cancer 2005; 116: 963–971.
5. Neugent AI: Cancer epidemiology and prevention. Sci Am 2004; 12: 2–11.
6. Roemer R, Taylor A, Lariviere J: Origins of the WHO framework convention on tobacco control. Am J Public Health 2005; 95: 936–938.
7. Yancik R: Population aging and cancer: A cross-national concern. Cancer J 2005; 11: 437–441.
8. Smith RA, Cokkinides V, Eyre HJ: American Cancer Society guidelines for the early detection of cancer, 2006. Cancer J Clin 2006; 56(1): 11–25.
9. Henschke CI: CT screening for lung cancer: update 2005. Surg Oncol Clin N Am 2005; 14: 761–776.
10. Mocharnuk RS: Controversies in Screening for early cancer detection. ASCO 2003 Special sessions; accessed February 2007 at: www.medscape.com/viewarticle/458140.

11. Jimbo M, Nease DE, Ruffin MT, et al: Information technology and cancer prevention. CA Cancer J Clin 2006; 56: 26–36.
12. Tsao AS, Kim ES, Hong WK: Chemoprevention of cancer. Cancer J Clin 2004; 54: 150–180.
13. Kelloff GJ, Lippman SM, Dannenberg AJ, et al: Progress in chemoprevention drug development: The promise of molecular biomarkers for prevention of intraepithelial neoplasia and cancer – a plan to move forward. Clin Cancer Res 2006; 12(12): 3661–3697.
14. Hanahan D, Weinberg RA: The hallmarks of cancer. Cell 2000; 100: 57–70.
15. Chen Y, Hunter DJ: Molecular epidemiology of cancer. Cancer J Clin 2005; 55(1): 45–54.
16. Ramaswamy S, Golub TR: DNA microarrays in clinical oncology. J Clin Oncol 2002; 20(7): 1932–1941.
17. Quackenbush J: Microarray analysis and tumor classification. N Engl J Med 2006; 354: 2463–2472.
18. Geho DH, Petricoin EF, Liotta LA: Blasting into the microworld of tissue proteomics: A new window on cancer. Clin Cancer Research 2004; 10: 825–827.
19. Smith L, Lind MJ, Welham KJ, et al: Cancer proteomics and its application to discovery of therapy response markers in human cancer. Cancer 2006; 107(2): 232–241.
20. Herbst RS, Bajorin DF, Bleiberg H, et al: Clinical cancer advances 2005: Major research advances in cancer treatment, prevention, and screening – a report from the American Society of Clinical Oncology. J Clin Oncol 2006; 24(1): 190–205.
21. Von Hoff DD, Gray PJ, Dragovich T: Pursuing therapeutic targets that are and are not there: A tumor's context of vulnerability. Semin Oncol 2006; 33(4): 367–368.
22. Ettinger DS, Bepler G, Bueno R, et al: Non-small cell lung cancer clinical practice guidelines in oncology. J Natl Compr Canc Netw 2006; 4(6): 548–582.

The role of molecular probes and other markers in the diagnosis and characterization of malignancy

2

Tad Wieczorek and Janina A. Longtine

Histopathological assessment is still the cornerstone in the diagnosis, classification and grading of malignancies. Light microscopic evaluation augmented by histochemical stains is sufficient in the majority of cases to provide adequate information for diagnosis and prognostication. However, it is limited by subjectivity and imprecision in the evaluation of poorly differentiated malignancies, tumours of unknown primary origin and unusual neoplasms. In an era of increasingly sophisticated therapeutic protocols (which sometimes target the molecular events leading to cancer) and the need to maximize information gained from minimally invasive samples (such as core biopsy or fine-needle aspiration), ancillary techniques have been developed to increase the specificity and reproducibility of diagnosis. These rely on cell-specific antigen expression and, more importantly, tumour-specific genetic changes that provide diagnostic, prognostic and/or therapeutic information.

In most instances, the advent of monoclonal antibodies directed against cellular proteins, coupled with the immunoperoxidase technique, has superseded direct ultrastructural evaluation in allowing more accurate designation of the epithelial, mesenchymal, haematolymphoid, neuroendocrine or glial origin of neoplasms. A cardinal example is immunolocalization of cytoskeletal intermediate filaments, which are differentially expressed in different cell types. Table 2.1 lists the intermediate filaments most useful in determining the cell lineage of tumours. The cytokeratins are a complex family of polypeptides that are expressed in various combinations in different epithelial cell types. Antibodies to cytokeratin subtypes can sometimes be utilized to identify the epithelial origin of a metastatic carcinoma of unknown primary site. For example, the pattern of reactivity for cytokeratin 7 (54 kD), which is expressed in most glandular and ductal epithelium and transitional epithelium of the urinary tract, and for cytokeratin 20 (46 kD), which is more restricted in its expression, has been helpful in this regard.[1]

In addition to the intermediate filaments, other monoclonal antibodies to cellular or tumour antigens are available. In the past decade, advances in the technique of immunohistochemistry have allowed

Table 2.1 Cytoskeletal intermediate filaments

Cell type	Intermediate filaments	Molecular weight or subtype	Presence in tumour
Epithelial	Cytokeratins	40–67	Keratinizing and non-keratinizing carcinomas
Mesenchymal	Vimentin	58	Wide distribution: sarcomas, melanomas, many lymphomas, some carcinomas
Muscle	Desmin	53	Leiomyosarcomas, rhabdomyosarcomas
Glial astrocytes	Glial fibrillary acidic protein	51	Gliomas (including astrocytomas), ependymomas
Neurons	Neurofilament proteins	68, 160, 200	Neural tumours, neuroblastomas

consistent, reliable application in routinely processed surgical pathology specimens.[2] Antigen retrieval techniques (including proteolytic digestion and heat-induced antigen retrieval), sensitive detection systems, automation and a broad range of antibodies have all contributed to this advance. Table 2.2 lists a panel of antibodies that can be utilized in routine formalin-fixed paraffin-embedded tissue to diagnose poorly differentiated neoplasms. A differential diagnosis is generated by clinical and morphological features, which can then be further refined by the use of immunohistochemistry. It is important to realize that the majority of antibodies are not entirely specific in lineage determination, and "aberrant" staining patterns are observed. In addition, there is biological variation in poorly differentiated neoplasms resulting in variation in protein expression. Therefore, accuracy is enhanced by using a panel of antisera to determine lineage or primary site. One application of this principle is distinguishing between poorly differentiated adenocarcinoma and mesothelioma in pleural tumours. Table 2.3 demonstrates the differential immunoprofile.

While a panel of monoclonal markers greatly aids in the diagnosis of a particular cancer, three malignancies can be confirmed solely by demonstrating the presence of a highly specific protein. Papillary and

Table 2.2 Immunocytochemistry in the differential diagnosis of malignancies

Malignancy	Keratin	Chromo-granin/ synaptophysin	S100	MART-1	LCA	OCT 3/4	SMA/ desmin
Carcinoma	+	–	–/+	–	–	–	–
Germ cell	+/–*	–	–	–	–	+/–	–
Lymphoma	–	–	–	–	+	–	–
Melanoma	–	–	+	+/–	–	–	–
Neuroendocrine	+/–	+	–	–	–	–	–
Sarcoma**	–/+	–	–/+	–/+	–	–	+/–

+ positive   +/– mainly positive, occasionally negative
– negative   –/+ mainly negative, occasionally positive

* Keratin is usually negative in seminomas, but positive in non-seminomatous germ cell tumours

**Sarcomas are a heterogeneous family of neoplasms and immunohistochemical staining patterns depend on the specific histological subtype

MART-1, Melanoma antigen recognized by T cells 1
LCA, Leukocyte common antigen
OCT3/4, Organic cation transporter 3/4
SMA, Smooth muscle actin

Table 2.3 Antibody panel in the differential diagnosis of adenocarcinoma and mesothelioma

Malignancy	Keratin*	WT-1	CD15 (Leu-M1)	CEA
Adenocarcinoma	+	–	+	+
Mesothelioma	+	+	–	–

*Keratin positivity in the appropriate clinicopathological setting limits the differential diagnosis to adenocarcinoma and mesothelioma

+ positive   – negative
CEA, carcinoembryonic antigen

follicular thyroid carcinomas are characterized by immunoreactivity to thyroglobulin, prostate carcinoma by detection of prostate-specific antigen, and breast carcinoma by a positive reaction for gross cystic disease fluid protein, which is present in approximately 50–70% of cases. It is noteworthy that the latter protein is also present in the rare apocrine gland carcinoma. Other antibodies which are not tissue-specific markers but useful in antibody panels include TTF-1 for pulmonary adenocarcinoma, RCC antigen for renal cell carcinoma, CD117 (c-kit) for gastrointestinal stromal tumours and CD31 (platelet endothelial cell adhesion molecule) for vascular endothelial neoplasms. Immunostains are also helpful in the delineation of normal tissue architecture and its abrogation in neoplasia. For example, immunostaining for p63 (a nuclear antigen expressed in myoepithelial cells of the breast and basal cells of the prostate) aids in the detection of ductal/glandular structures without the normal myoepithelial framework, the hallmark of invasive neoplasia.

While the cellular proteins expressed in particular types of neoplasia are fundamental to their diagnostic characterization, somatic mutations (i.e. mutations that occur in the genes of non-germline tissues) are central to the development of cancer. A series of different mutations in critical genes is probably necessary for malignant transformation to occur. The mutations may be deletions, duplications, point mutations and/or chromosomal translocations in the DNA of the tumour precursor cell. The mutations affect regulation of the cell cycle, differentiation, apoptosis, or cell–cell and cell–matrix interactions. Different neoplasms have different combinations of genetic alterations, which lead to clonal proliferations of cells. These genetic alterations, although fundamental in tumour biology, can also be used as diagnostic or prognostic markers for malignancies. This is best characterized in lymphomas and leukaemias where specific genetic translocations result in the production of chimeric mRNA and novel proteins. These translocations are the *sine qua non* for the classification of some leukaemias, such as the Philadelphia chromosome t(9;22)(q34;q11) for chronic myelogenous leukaemia and t(15;17)(q22;q11-21) for acute promyelocytic leukaemia.[3] Single nucleotide mutations may also be important in haematopoietic neoplasia; for example the *JAK2* V617F mutation is frequently present in chronic myeloproliferative disorders.[4] While genetic alterations in carcinomas are more complex than single point mutations or chromosome translocations, simple chromosomal translocations also commonly occur in (and characterize) soft tissue tumours.[5,6]

A global assessment of structural cytogenetic changes in a neoplasm is provided by full karyotypic analysis, which requires fresh, viable tumour. By contrast, fluorescence *in situ* hybridization (FISH) is a more targeted approach that can be performed on interphase nuclei obtained from frozen or fixed paraffin-embedded tissue and can identify specific characteristic cytogenetic abnormalities as an adjunct to tumour diagnosis. For example, FISH probes that flank the *EWS* gene region show a "split apart" signal when an *EWS* rearrangement is present, as in Ewing's sarcoma (see Figure 2.1). In addition, many of the characteristic cytogenetic abnormalities of neoplasms have been cloned and sequenced allowing for the utilization of molecular biology techniques such as Southern blot hybridization or, more commonly, the polymerase chain reaction (PCR). These techniques utilize fresh or frozen tumour, or even fixed, embedded tissue (with PCR), and improve diagnoses by identifying the characteristic chromosomal translocations of malignancies at the molecular level. With PCR, a specific translocation can be detected in as little as 1 in 100,000 or 1 in 1,000,000 cells as compared with 1 in 100 for FISH analysis. Thus, PCR provides a sensitive method for diagnosis and for monitoring response to therapy. For example, the t(9;22)(q34:q11) of chronic myelogenous leukaemia juxtaposes the *BCR* and *ABL1* genes resulting in a unique chimeric mRNA that can be detected by a quantitative real-time RT-PCR technique. Peripheral blood cell RNA is converted to cDNA by reverse transcription (RT). The resultant *BCR-ABL1* cDNA is quantified by monitoring fluorescently labelled oligonucleotide probes that specifically hybridize with the target during each cycle of PCR amplification (see Figure 2.2). Clinical trials with the tyrosine kinase inhibitor imatinib

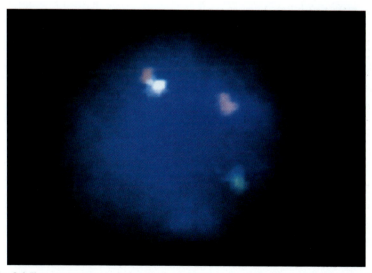

Fig. 2.1 Fluorescence *in situ* hybridization (FISH) on a sample obtained by fine-needle aspiration shows an interphase nucleus with red and green probes flanking each of two copies of the *EWS* gene, demonstrating one fused and one split signal. The split signal indicates rearrangement of the *EWS* gene region. (Courtesy of Dr. Paola Dal Cin, Cytogenetics Laboratory, Brigham and Women's Hospital.)

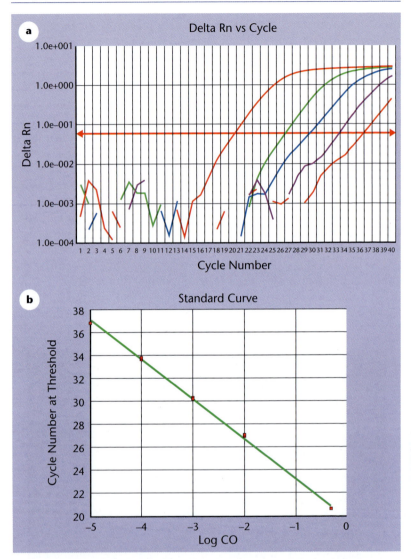

Fig. 2.2 (a) "Taq-Man^{TM}" (Applied Biosystems) quantitative RT-PCR results for dilutions (1:1, 10^{-2}, 10^{-3}, 10^{-4}, 10^{-5}) of K562 cell line RNA which express chimeric *BCR-ABL1* mRNA. After approximately 15 cycles of PCR, the sample with the most *BCR-ABL1* mRNA (1:1) enters the linear phase of exponential amplification as measured by fluorescence accumulation monitored in real time. Samples with less target require more PCR cycles to reach the exponential phase. **(b)** For quantitation, a standard curve is generated plotting the PCR cycle number at threshold (red line in middle of exponential phase) against log concentration of target. Unknown samples can be quantified by plotting against the standard curve.

defined a target of a minimal residual level of *BCR-ABL1* RNA transcripts that is associated with progression-free survival (see Figure 2.3).[7,8] Rising levels of *BCR-ABL1* mRNA in patients on tyrosine kinase inhibitors or status post transplantation are indicative of a molecular relapse and the need for alternate or additional therapy. Southern blot hybridization or PCR can also identify clonal rearrangements of the immunoglobulin or T-cell receptor genes as an adjunct to the diagnosis of lymphoma or lymphoid leukaemias (see Figure 2.4).

Genetic analysis of neoplasms may also provide prognostic information, such as identifying the *BCR-ABL1* rearrangement in Philadelphia chromosome-positive acute lymphoblastic leukaemia (ALL) or *N-MYC* amplification in neuroblastoma. In addition, genetic analysis is playing an increasing role in therapeutic planning, as therapies tailored to specific genetic "lesions" are developed. Examples of such lesions include *HER2* amplification in breast cancer[9] and the epidermal growth factor receptor gene (*EGFR*) mutation in lung cancer.[10,11] These genetic lesions

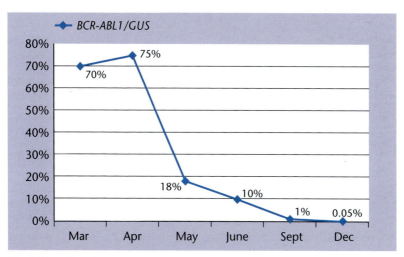

Fig. 2.3 Timeline of response to the tyrosine kinase inhibitor imatinib as monitored by real-time RT-PCR analysis of *BCR-ABL1* mRNA expressed as a ratio to the normalizing gene, *GUS*. Patients who achieve a 3-log reduction of transcript level by 12 months of therapy have a negligible risk of disease progression in the following 12 months.[8]

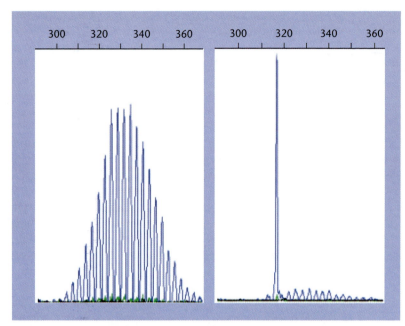

Fig. 2.4 Polymerase chain reaction (PCR) amplification of the immunoglobulin heavy chain (IgH) gene with primers to the variable and joining regions that flank the unique IgH gene rearrangement of B-cells. B-cell IgH rearrangements differ by size and sequence. Fluorescent primers are incorporated into the PCR product, which are then analyzed by capillary gel electrophoresis. (**a**) The Gaussian distribution of a polyclonal population of B cells. (**b**) A dominant peak of 318 bp representing a monoclonal population in a B-cell lymphoma.

may be detected either by evaluation of aberrant protein expression (as in immunohistochemical detection of membranous overexpression of HER2 oncoprotein in breast cancer), by gene amplification (as in FISH analysis of *HER2*), or by molecular testing (as in *EGFR* point or small deletion mutation analysis in lung cancer, see Figure 2.5). Quantification of the expression levels of large numbers of genes in specific types of neoplasia by oligonucleotide chips or cDNA microarrays, "expression profiling", has led to the identification of subsets of genes that provide prognostic information, such as in diffuse large B-cell lymphoma (see Figure 2.6).[12] It has even become feasible to measure the expression level of multiple genes (by RT-PCR) in routinely prepared, paraffin-embedded tumour samples, as in the multigene assay to

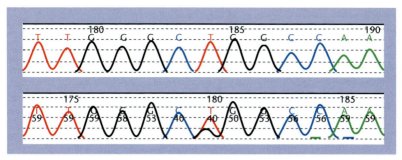

Fig. 2.5 Lung adenocarcinoma DNA sequence analysis of exon 21 of the *EGFR* receptor gene. The top row shows normal or wildtype exon sequence. The bottom row shows the heterozygous T to C point mutation, which characterizes the L858R mutation, a common mutation in carcinomas responsive to tyrosine kinase inhibitors.

predict recurrence of tamoxifen-treated, node-negative breast cancer.[13] This assay measures the expression level of genes involved in key aspects of tumour biology such as proliferation, invasion and oestrogen response and its quantitative result has potential application in therapeutic planning. As key genes (and hence proteins) are identified by expression profiling, expression can be assayed by routine immunohistochemistry. An important and practical example of this strategy was the development of a specific antibody to P504S (AMACR/racemase), a protein product strongly expressed in prostatic adenocarcinoma and prostatic intraepithelial neoplasia, but typically not in benign prostatic epithelium.[14] This immunostain is therefore useful in supporting a diagnosis of prostatic adenocarcinoma in cases where the morphological findings are subtle – as in the diagnosis of minimal adenocarcinoma on needle biopsy.

The genetics of cancer also extends to inherited predisposition to neoplasms described in a number of families.[15] These syndromes include germline mutations of tumour suppressor genes, such as familial retinoblastoma, and mutations of DNA repair genes as in ataxia-telangectasia or hereditary non-polyposis colon cancer. Some of these are listed in Table 2.4.

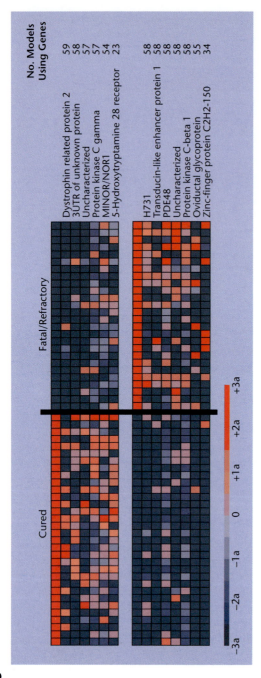

Fig. 2.6 Genes included in the DLBCL outcome model. Genes expressed at higher levels in cured disease are listed on top and those that were more abundant in fatal disease are shown on the bottom. Red indicates high expression; blue, low expression. Colour scale at bottom indicates relative expression in standard deviations from the mean. Each column is a sample, each row is a gene. Expression profiles of the 32 cured DLBCLs are on the left; profiles of the fatal/refractory tumours are on the right. Models with the highest accuracy were obtained using 13 genes. Reproduced by permission from Macmillan Publishers Ltd: Nature Medicine. Shipp M, Ross K, Tamayo P, et al: Diffuse large B-cell lymphoma outcome prediction by gene expression profiling and supervised machine learning. Nature Med 2002; 8: 68–74. © 2002.

Table 2.4 Examples of inherited syndromes predisposing to cancer

Syndrome	Chromosome locus	Gene
Ataxia-telangiactasia	11q22	*ATM*
Hereditary breast/ovarian cancer	17q21 13q12	*BRCA1* *BRCA2*
Familial adenomatous polyposis	5q21-q22	*APC*
Familial retinoblastoma	13q14	*RB1*
Hereditary non-polyposis colorectal cancer (Lynch syndrome)	2p22-p21 3p21 2q31-q33 7p22	*MSH2* *MLH1* *PMS1* *PMS2*
Li-Fraumeni	17p13	*TP53*
Multiple endocrine neoplasia, Type 1	11q13	*MEN1*
Multiple endocrine neoplasia, Type 2	10q11.2	*RET*
Neurofibromatosis, Type 1	17q11	*NF1*
Neurofibromatosis, Type 2	22q12	*NF2*
von Hippel-Lindau disease	3p26-p25	*VHL*

REFERENCES

1. Chu P, Wu E, Weiss LM: Cytokeratin 7 and cytokeratin 20 expression in epithelial neoplasms: a survey of 435 cases. Mod Pathol 2000; 13(9): 962–971.
2. Chan JKC: Advances in immunohistochemistry: Impact on surgical pathology practice. Seminars Diagn Pathol 2000; 17: 170–177.
3. Jaffe ES, Stein HN, Vardiman JW, eds: World Health Organization Classification of Tumours, Pathology and Genetics of Tumours of Haematopoietic and Lymphoid Tissues. IARC Press, Lyon, 2001.
4. Percy MJ, McMullin MF: The V617F JAK2 mutation and the myeloproliferative disorders. Hematol Oncol 2005; 23(3-4): 91–93.
5. Sandberg AA: Cytogenetics and molecular genetics of bone and soft-tissue tumors. Am J Med Genet 2002; 115(3): 189–193.
6. Antonescu CR: The role of genetic testing in soft tissue sarcoma. Histopathology 2006; 48(1): 13–21.
7. O'Brien SG, Guilhot F, Larson RA, et al: Imatinib compared with interferon and low-dose cytarabine for newly diagnosed chronic-phase chronic myeloid leukemia. N Engl J Med 2003; 348: 994–1004.
8. Hughes TP, Kaeda J, Branford S, et al: Frequency of major molecular responses to imatinib or interferon alfa plus cytarabine in newly diagnosed chronic myeloid leukemia. N Engl J Med 2003; 349: 1423–1432.

9. Slamon DJ, Leyland-Jones B, Shak S, et al: Use of chemotherapy plus a monoclonal antibody against HER2 for metastatic breast cancer that overexpresses HER2. N Engl J Med 2001; 344: 783–792.

10. Lynch TJ, Bell DW, Sordella R, et al: Activating mutations in the epidermal growth factor receptor underlying responsiveness of non-small-cell lung cancer to gefitinib. N Engl J Med 2004; 350: 2129–2139.

11. Paez JG, Janne PA, Lee JC, et al: EGFR mutations in lung cancer: correlation with clinical response to gefitinib therapy. Science 2004; 304: 1497–1500.

12. Shipp M, Ross K, Tamayo P, et al: Diffuse large B-cell lymphoma outcome prediction by gene expression profiling and supervised machine learning. Nature Med 2002; 8: 68–74.

13. Paik S, Shak S, Tang G, et al: A multigene assay to predict recurrence of tamoxifen-treated, node-negative breast cancer. N Engl J Med 2004; 351: 2817–2826.

14. Beach R, Gown AM, De Peralta-Venturina MN, et al: P504S immunohistochemical detection in 405 prostatic specimens including 376 18-gauge needle biopsies. Am J Surg Pathol 2002; 26(12): 1588–1596.

15. Scriver CR, Beaudet AL, Sly WS, Valle D, eds: Metabolic and Molecular Bases of Inherited Disease, 8th edn. McGraw-Hill, New York, 2001.

Lung cancer: aetiology, histopathology and clinical manifestations

3

Ravi Salgia, Ramon Blanco, Arthur T. Skarin and Christopher S. Lathan

INCIDENCE AND AETIOLOGY

Lung cancer is the most common cancer in the world with about 1.2 million new cases diagnosed per year.[1] The American Cancer Society estimated that there would be 114,760 new cases in men and 98,620 new cases in women in 2006.[2] Lung cancer will still be the leading cause of death from malignancy in both sexes in the US in 2007, resulting in an estimated 70,880 deaths in women and 89,510 deaths in men.[2] Lung cancer is responsible for more deaths than breast, colon and prostate cancers added together. The vast majority of cases (85% or more) are due to cigarette smoking. Other aetiological factors include asbestos (shipyard workers, insulation workers), radon gas (underground mining), ionizing radiation and certain industrial agents and compounds (chloromethyl ether, arsenic, nickel-cadmium and chromium). Tobacco smoking is thought to be synergistic with many of these carcinogens.

Whereas lung cancer is one of the easiest cancers to prevent, it is one of the most difficult to cure, owing to the fact that the majority of patients present with locally advanced or metastatic disease that responds poorly to systemic therapy. The 5-year survival rate for all patients is about 15%, although survival is clearly related to stage at presentation. If a patient survives the initial cancer, the risk of a subsequent lung cancer increases to 3–5% per year. By discontinuing cigarette smoking, the patient lowers the risk for primary lung cancer as well as subsequent cancer, but it takes 15–20 years before the risk approaches that of non-smokers; the residual risk is influenced by the age at stopping smoking.[3] Passive smoking accounts for 3–5% of all cases of lung cancer and appears to be increasing. According to the Surgeon General in the US, 5000–10,000 of the deaths due to lung cancer each year occur in patients exposed to second-hand smoke.

LUNG CANCER, GENDER AND AGE

Lung cancer rates in women have risen dramatically, both worldwide and in the US. Population-based data by the National Cancer Institute

Surveillance, Epidemiology and End Results (SEER) Program have shown that the age-adjusted rate for lung cancer for all race/sex groups has risen sharply since 1950. The incidence started rising in the mid-1930s and overtook breast cancer as the leading cause of cancer deaths among women in the late 1980s. This observation correlates with the increase in the number of women who smoke. The male to female ratio is 3.47 in patients over 45 years of age and 1.7 in patients younger than 45 years.

HISTOPATHOLOGY

Over 95% of primary lung neoplasms are of epithelial origin (carcinomas), comprising four main types (see Table 3.1). Based on clinical features and biological properties, these carcinomas can be separated into two major categories: non-small cell lung cancer (NSCLC; squamous cell, adenocarcinoma and undifferentiated large cell types) and small cell lung cancer.[4] About 5% of lung cancers are composed of rare mixed epithelial types or neoplasms arising from bronchial glands and other tissues (see Table 3.1).

PREINVASIVE LESIONS

In the World Health Organization (WHO)/International Association for the Study of Lung Cancer 1999 classification, preinvasive lesions include squamous dysplasia/carcinoma *in situ* (leading to squamous cell carcinoma), atypical adenomatous hyperplasia (AAH, characterized by discrete ill-defined bronchioloalveolar proliferation, leading to adenocarcinoma) and diffuse idiopathic pulmonary neuroendocrine cell hyperplasia (DIPNECH, characterized by proliferation of neuroendocrine cells throughout the peripheral airways, leading to carcinoid).[5]

NON-SMALL CELL LUNG CANCER

NSCLC comprises about 75% of all lung cancers. They are subdivided into three groups. Squamous cell carcinoma is characterized by keratin formation (cytokeratin proteins are intermediate filaments). Keratin may appear under the light microscope as 'keratin pearls' (see Figure 3.3) or as desmosomes (a type of tight junction seen as 'intercellular bridges'). The incidence of this type of lung cancer is decreasing in the US for unknown reasons, but perhaps related to the introduction of stronger cigarette filters that remove large particles. Most squamous cell carcinomas arise from the central or proximal tracheal-bronchial tree in areas of squamous cell

Table 3.1 Pathology of lung malignancies and associated clinical features

Type[x]	Relative incidence (%)	Major location	Associated clinical or paraneoplastic syndrome*
Non-small cell lung cancer	75		
Adenocarcinoma	35–40[+]	Peripheral	Hypertrophic osteoarthropathy
Bronchioloalveolar cell carcinoma (BAC)	5[+]	Peripheral	Voluminous watery sputum
Mixed adeno-squamous	2		
Squamous	25–30[++]	Central	Hypercalcaemia
Large cell	8	Peripheral	Gynaecomastia, galactorrhoea
Small cell lung cancer	15[++]	Central	SIADH, Cushing's syndrome, Eaton-Lambert syndrome, hypocalcaemia
Combined cell type	<5		
Miscellaneous	5–10		
Mesothelioma	1–2[+]	Pleural	Hypoglycaemia
Carcinoid[+++]	1	Peripheral/ central	Vasomotor symptoms
Sarcomatoid carcinoma[++++]	1	Peripheral/ central	Metastasis as epithelial or sarcomatous elements
Mucoepidermoid	1	Central	Is usually low-grade
Adenoid cystic carcinoma	1	Central	Long natural history, tendency to spread along nerve tracts
Mesenchymal tumours[xx]	1	Peripheral/ central	Prognosis is variable
Lymphoproliferative tumours	2	Peripheral/ central	Autoimmune phenomenon

[x]Modified from Travis, et al, WHO 2004
*May vary among cell types
[+]Incidence increasing
[++]Incidence decreasing
[+++]Typical and atypical
[++++]Includes spindle cell, giant cell, carcinosarcoma, pulmonary blastoma
[xx]Includes angiosarcoma, others
SIADH, syndrome of inappropriate antidiuretic hormone secretion

metaplasia, dysplasia and carcinoma *in situ*. Squamous cell carcinomas grow relatively slowly, and tend to cavitate in about 20% of cases. About one-third of squamous cell carcinomas are poorly differentiated and show a greater potential for metastatic spread. Poorly differentiated squamous cell carcinomas may acquire a spindle cell morphology that may mimic a sarcoma; identification of such tumours is based on finding a transition zone between the epithelial-appearing tumour cells and the spindle cells and/or on the demonstration of keratin in the spindle cells by immuno-histochemistry.

Adenocarcinoma is characterized by gland formation (well and moderately differentiated) or by the presence of mucin production in a solid tumour (poorly differentiated) as determined by mucin stains (mucicarmine and D-PAS) (see Figure 3.5). Adenocarcinomas are increasing in frequency in the US and Europe: at most medical centres in the US, they are now more common than squamous cell carcinomas, although the reverse is seen in Europe. Alterations in cigarette smoking and the design of improved cigarette filters has been implicated in this change.[6] In about two-thirds of cases, adenocarcinomas originate in peripheral airways and alveoli. Classically, they were thought to arise from scars ('scar carcinoma'). This view is no longer accepted: the 'scar tissue' (desmoplasia) is now thought to be induced by the neoplastic cells. Around one-third of cases arise centrally, in larger bronchi, from either the surface epithelium or the submucosal glands. Peripheral adenocarcinomas frequently present as subpleural nodules, often with a malignant pleural effusion. These cases must be differentiated by means of special stains from malignant mesothelioma, which lacks mucin. Metastases from adenocarcinoma to distant sites occur early (e.g. before symptoms or diagnosis) in many patients. Adenocarcinoma arising from sites other than lung can also look very similar to adenocarcinoma arising in the lung. Cytokeratins (7 versus 20) can aid in distinguishing adenocarcinoma from lung versus that from other sites (in the case of lung, cytokeratin 7 is usually positive and cytokeratin 20 usually negative). Thyroid transcription factor-1 (TTF-1), is found almost exclusively in adenocarcinoma of the lung and thyroid cancer and is useful in the differential diagnosis of metastatic adenocarcinoma from an unknown primary site.[7]

Bronchioloalveolar carcinoma (BAC) is a subtype of well-differentiated adenocarcinoma, constituting about 3% of cases, and is increasing in frequency. It is the one subtype of lung carcinoma (in addition to carcinoid tumours) that is not significantly associated with cigarette smoking. BAC arises from the peripheral bronchioles or alveoli. About 50% are mucin-secreting tumours consisting of tall columnar cells, whereas the remaining 50% have little or no mucin and consist of peg-shaped ('hobnail') cells with variable degrees of pleomorphism. They are thought to arise from Clara cells or type II pneumocytes. Some adenocarcinomas may contain a small proportion of tumour cells with BAC morphology, typically in the periphery of the tumour. In the WHO classification, true BAC has growth in a lepidic fashion with lack of invasive growth.[5] BAC tends to spread throughout air passages, while preserving (or recapitulating) the septal and lobular architecture. The tumour is slow growing and usually metastasizes late in the course of the disease. It characteristically induces a voluminous clear sputum production (bronchorrhoea). Prognosis is related to stage of disease, but because BAC may be mistaken for chronic infection or diffuse interstitial disease, there may be a long delay in diagnosis. Previous studies indicated that BAC responded poorly to treatment and carried a worse prognosis than other NSCLC subtypes, but recent data have not supported this premise. In contrast, the activity of epithelial growth factor receptor inhibitors has caused increased interest in this clinical subtype.[8]

Undifferentiated large cell carcinoma is characterized by large cells with vesicular nuclei, prominent eosinophilic nucleoli, moderate-to-abundant cytoplasm, distinct cytoplasmic membrane and no evidence of squamous or glandular differentiation by light microscopy. Some of these tumours may contain features of either squamous and/or glandular differentiation as evidenced by immunohistochemistry or electron microscopy, implying some heterogeneity in this group. Giant cell and clear cell variants are uncommon. A giant cell variant may mimic an anaplastic large cell lymphoma (Ki-1 positive or large T-cell lymphoma). Clinically, most patients with large cell carcinoma present with large, bulky, peripheral tumours. Metastases occur early, and the overall 5-year survival is under 5%.

SMALL CELL LUNG CANCER

Small cell lung cancer (SCLC) represents about 15% of all lung cancers, is extremely aggressive, is frequently associated with distant metastases and has the poorest prognosis of all primary lung neoplasms. SCLC has a central origin in most cases, although 10% of these tumours are found in the peripheral lung field. The tumour often has a white-tan appearance, is friable and shows extensive necrosis. Histologically, they are characterized by scant cytoplasm or a high nuclear:cytoplasmic ratio, fine chromatin and 'nuclear molding'. Small cells are characterized as 'small blue cell tumour' and need to be distinguished from lymphoma, carcinoid tumours, Ewing's sarcoma and peripheral neuroectodermal tumours. The rapid growth and scanty cytoplasm of small cell carcinomas make them unusually susceptible to ischaemic necrosis, as well as crush artefact, during handling and fixation. Although not pathognomonic, the so-called Azzopardi effect (crushed DNA material encrusted around blood vessels) is very characteristic (see Figure 3.13c). The subclassification of small cell carcinoma into oat cell, intermediate cell and combined oat cell carcinoma has been dropped from the new WHO classification. Approximately 10% of SCLC are combined with NSCLC components (with large cells 4–6%, 1–3% with adenocarcinoma or squamous cell carcinoma).

Most (but not all) small cell carcinomas contain dense-core granules (containing amines, peptide products, L-dopa decarboxylase), indicating neuroendocrine differentiation. Immunohistochemical studies demonstrate the presence of neurone-specific enolase (NSE), chromogranin A, Leu-7 (a natural killer cell antigen also present in other neuroendocrine cells) and synaptophysin. Other antigens that may also be expressed are carcinoembryonic antigen (CEA), adrenocorticotrophin hormone (ACTH) and 'big' ACTH. SCLC cells, as with most carcinomas, express keratin proteins. Small cell carcinomas produce and release into the circulation a variety of functioning polypeptide hormones that can result in paraneoplastic syndromes. They also grow in a submucosal pattern with a high frequency of lymphatic and vascular invasion. Prominent mediastinal adenopathy is often present. Approximately 70% of patients have metastatic disease at the time of diagnosis. Almost any organ can be involved, but preferential sites include the liver, bone, bone marrow, CNS, adrenal glands, abdominal lymph nodes, pancreas, skin and endocrine organs.

CARCINOID TUMOUR AND THE SPECTRUM OF NEUROENDOCRINE TUMOURS OF THE LUNG

The classification of neuroendocrine neoplasms of the lung has evolved substantially over the past two decades. There is a spectrum of tumour types ranging from carcinoid tumour through atypical carcinoid, large cell neuroendocrine carcinoma to small cell lung cancer, that have different morphological appearances and substantially different clinical behaviour. Typical carcinoid (TC) or carcinoid tumours (bronchial carcinoid tumours) are similar to tumours arising in the gastrointestinal tract and elsewhere. They are characterized by small (0.7–3.5 cm), well-circumscribed solid tan-yellow nodules with no necrosis or haemorrhage. Usually they are located centrally. By light microscopy, tumour cells are round, uniform in size, with finely granular eosinophilic cytoplasm. The nucleus is centrally placed with finely granular or stippled chromatin and small nucleoli. The cells arrange themselves in an organoid pattern (cords, nests and acini may be formed). Mitoses are rare and necrosis is not seen. By electron microscopy numerous cytoplasmic membrane-bound, dense-core granules (90–450 nm) are usually seen. By immunohistology they are usually positive for NSE, chromogranin A, Leu-7, synaptophysin, bombesin, CEA, ACTH, calcitonin and keratin. Carcinoid tumours may be responsible for ectopic hormone secretion, particularly 5-hydroxytryptamine, ACTH, vasopressin and insulin. Typical carcinoids have low malignant potential. Atypical carcinoid (AC) is similar to TC, but the cells are usually larger, contain foci of necrosis, and mitoses are seen (usually 3–4/10 HPF). Atypical carcinoids can follow a more aggressive clinical course than TC and have metastatic potential. AC represent approximately 10% of all carcinoid tumours.

Large cell neuroendocrine carcinoma (LCNEC) is a malignant neuroendocrine neoplasm composed of large polygonal cells with a relatively low nuclear:cytoplasmic ratio, coarse nuclear chromatin, frequent nucleoli, high mitotic rate (>10/10 HPF) and frequent necrosis.[9] The cells in LCNEC are larger than cells in SCLC and have more abundant eosinophilic cytoplasm.

CHROMOSOMES, GENES AND LUNG CANCER

The evolution of normal cells to cancer is currently understood as a multistep process. Insight into this evolution has been gained through recent advances in cytogenetics and cell biology but mainly through developments in molecular biology. It has become apparent that mutations in a limited number of genes, which control cell proliferation and differentiation, are key events in this process. Proto-oncogenes and tumour suppressor genes play major roles in malignant transformation of cells. Full discussion of this important topic is beyond the scope of this review. Readers are referred to detailed reviews.[4,10] One topic of therapeutic importance is the epidermal growth factor receptor present on the malignant cell in many patients with lung cancer.[11,12]

CLINICAL MANIFESTATIONS

The signs and symptoms of lung cancer may be related directly to the local effects of the primary malignancy, e.g. invasion of thoracic structures, or to distant metastases. Indirect signs and symptoms – para-neoplastic syndromes – may also be encountered as a result of the secretion of biologically active peptides and hormones, or as a result of tumour-related immune events (e.g. immune-mediated glomerulonephritis, neurological syndromes, etc.) (see Table 3.1).

Manifestations of early thoracic disease depend on the location of the primary cancer. Central (proximal) lesions often erode the bronchus and bronchial vessels, causing haemoptysis and cough. As the tumour spreads, bronchial obstruction with atelectasis and pneumonia may occur. Hilar adenopathy and cavitation of the primary cancer may also develop. Although small cell cancers are central in origin, they grow submucosally and less commonly cause haemoptysis. Due to lymphatic invasion, mediastinal adenopathy occurs in most cases. Compression of the recurrent laryngeal nerve results in hoarseness. Stridor may result from compression or invasion of the trachea or major bronchus. Invasion or compression of the superior vena cava leads to the so-called SVC syndrome. Extension of malignancy into the pericardium may result in pericardial effusion and in some cases acute cardiac tamponade.

Tumours arising in the periphery of the lung may cause chest pain and cough due to involvement of the pleura, often with malignant pleural effusion and resultant dyspnoea. Cancers arising in the apex of the lung grow into the adjacent soft tissues, resulting in a Pancoast tumour or superior sulcus tumour syndrome, the features of which may vary. The advanced syndrome is marked by shoulder pain radiating to the ulnar nerve distribution, rib and vertebral body destruction and Horner's syndrome (enophthalmos, ptosis, myosis and ipsilateral loss of sweating) due to invasion of the sympathetic nerves. With early involvement, mydriasis (pupillary dilatation) may be the first clue. Histologically, Pancoast tumours are usually squamous cell carcinomas, although other non-small cell types of cancer can occur. Unilateral supraclavicular adenopathy is a sign of advanced local disease.

Metastatic disease can occur to any organ and thus a variety of clinical and laboratory manifestations may be encountered. At autopsy, the frequency of extrathoracic metastases related to histological type of lung cancer is as follows: squamous cell carcinoma, 25–54%; adenocarcinoma, 50–82%; large cell carcinoma, 48–86%; and small cell carcinoma, 74–96%. Indirect manifestations of lung cancer vary from severe weight loss and cachexia, seen in up to one-third of patients, to one or more of several paraneoplastic syndromes. The latter are due to the secretion of biologically active peptides or hormones, immune-mediated manifestations or to unknown factors often related to certain histological cell types (see Table 3.5). Initial symptoms may be non-specific and result in delayed diagnosis. Hypertrophic osteoarthropathy can occur with symptoms of swelling and pain in the joints and extremities, and may be misdiagnosed as an inflammatory arthritis.

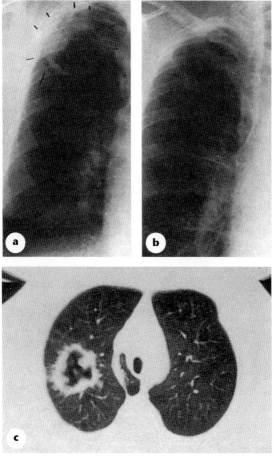

Fig. 3.1 Squamous cell carcinoma. A 58-year-old man who presented with increasing cough was found to have a large cavitating lesion in the right upper lung (a). (b) Chest film obtained 4 years earlier shows a small nodule that most likely represents the primary cancer. (c) Computed tomography scan shows a localized cavitating lesion. Squamous cell carcinoma often presents with cavitation due to tumour necrosis.

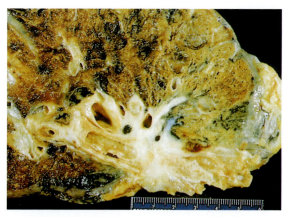

Fig. 3.2 Squamous cell carcinoma. A 66-year-old woman had a long-standing history of cigarette smoking and presented with metastatic disease. Bronchoscopy was positive for squamous cell carcinoma. Death resulted from widespread metastases. Mid-coronal section of the left lung shows local invasion of the large bronchi and hilum. Most squamous cell lung tumours are of central origin. (Courtesy of Pathology Department, Brigham and Women's Hospital, Boston, MA.)

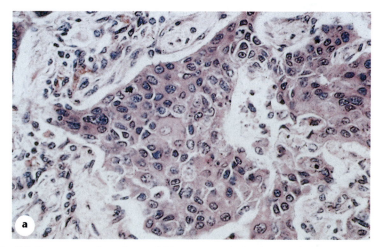

Fig. 3.3 Squamous cell carcinoma (**a**) Low-power photomicrograph shows an invasive squamous cell carcinoma. Note the distinction between the cells at the periphery and the keratinized cells in the centre of the island of tumour.

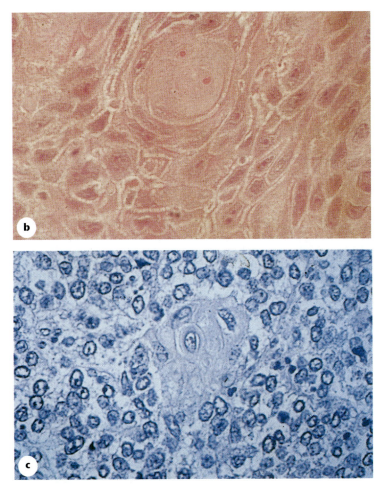

(b) This high-power view exhibits the classic appearance of a keratin pearl and intercellular bridges diagnostic for squamous cell carcinoma. (c) This poorly differentiated tumour shows a focal central keratinized area. Immunoperoxidase staining for keratin protein was positive (not shown).

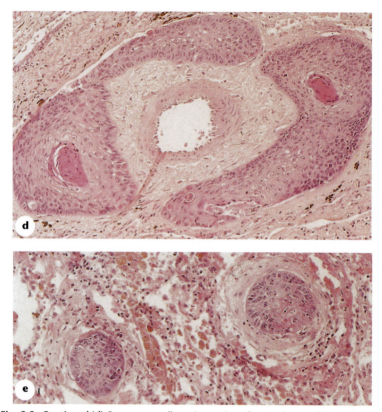

Fig. 3.3 *Continued* (d) Squamous cell carcinoma invading and extending through lymphatic vessels surrounding a small blood vessel. (e) Squamous cell carcinoma in blood vessels.

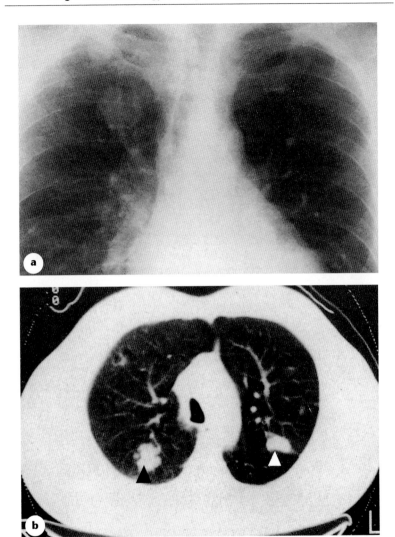

Fig. 3.4 Adenocarcinoma. (a) On routine medical examination, the chest film of a 64-year-old man shows bilateral primary lung tumours in the upper lobes; the lesion on the left side is partly obscured by the clavicle. (b) Computed tomography scan clearly defines the irregularly shaped primary lesions (arrows). Synchronous primary lung cancers occur in about 3–5% of patients and can be of different histological subgroups.

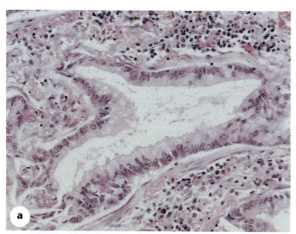

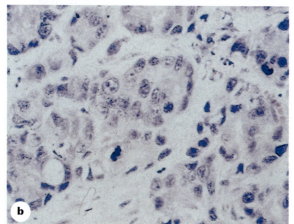

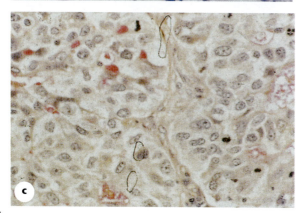

Fig. 3.5
Adenocarcinoma. (**a**) Microscopic section shows the typical appearance of a gland formation. (**b**) On high-power view, this poorly to moderately differentiated adenocarcinoma exhibits clusters of cells with eccentric nuclei and abundant cytoplasm. Note a cluster of tumour cells with a central lumen in the lower left of the field. (**c**) This poorly differentiated adenocarcinoma shows positive mucicarmine staining for intra- and extracytoplasmic mucin.

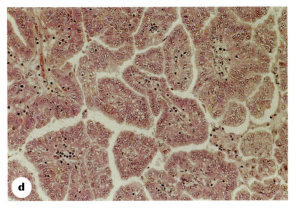

(d) Papillary adenocarcinoma of lung. Low-power view of a moderately well-differentiated adenocarcinoma with papillary features. Metastases from ovary, thyroid, breast or kidney cancer should be considered in the differential diagnosis of papillary adenocarcinoma.

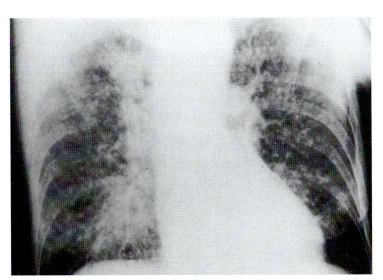

Fig. 3.6 Bronchioloalveolar carcinoma. A 60-year-old female presented with the classic features of advanced disease: increasing dyspnoea on exertion with a frequent cough that produced large amounts of frothy sputum. Chest radiograph shows extensive metastases throughout the lung fields with hilar and mediastinal adenopathy.

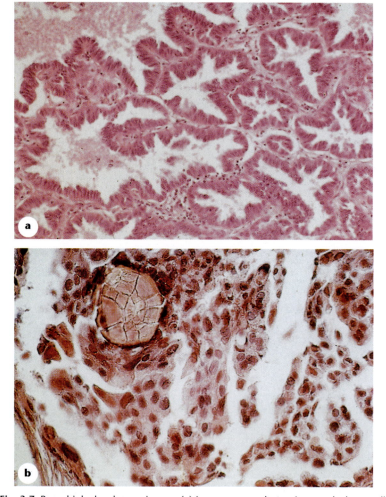

Fig. 3.7 Bronchioloalveolar carcinoma. (**a**) Lower-power photomicrograph shows tall columnar peg-shaped cells growing in a 'picket-fence' pattern on the alveolar walls. (**b**) On high-power view, a typical psammoma body, characterized by concentric laminations, is evident.

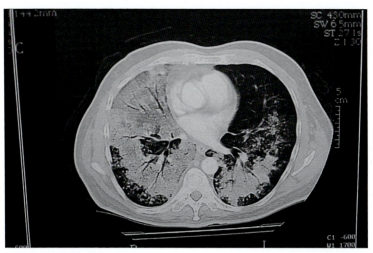

Fig. 3.8 Bronchioloalveolar carcinoma. Computed tomography scan shows bilateral lung lesions in this 48-year-old woman with cough and excessive sputum production. Note the classic air bronchograms.

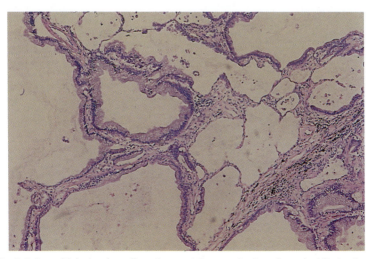

Fig. 3.9 Bronchioloalveolar cell carcinoma. Microscopic view shows lepidic (scale-like) growth along alveolar septa.

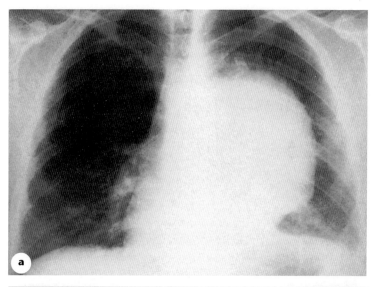

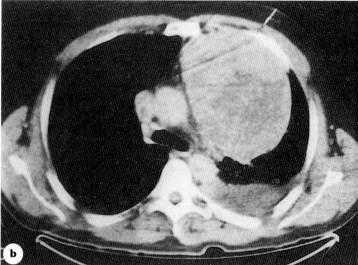

Fig. 3.10 Large cell carcinoma. A 45-year-old man with a history of chronic cigarette smoking developed increasing chest pain and cough. (**a**) Radiograph shows a huge primary mass. (**b**) Computed tomography scan shows the mass extending into the left anterior chest wall; a small pleural effusion is also apparent. Note the biopsy needle.

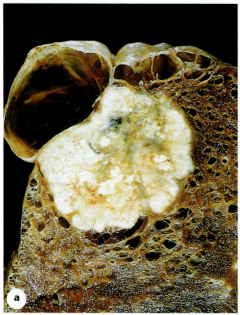

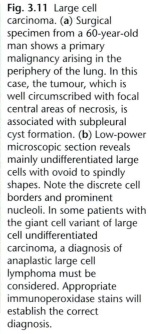

Fig. 3.11 Large cell carcinoma. (a) Surgical specimen from a 60-year-old man shows a primary malignancy arising in the periphery of the lung. In this case, the tumour, which is well circumscribed with focal central areas of necrosis, is associated with subpleural cyst formation. (b) Low-power microscopic section reveals mainly undifferentiated large cells with ovoid to spindly shapes. Note the discrete cell borders and prominent nucleoli. In some patients with the giant cell variant of large cell undifferentiated carcinoma, a diagnosis of anaplastic large cell lymphoma must be considered. Appropriate immunoperoxidase stains will establish the correct diagnosis.

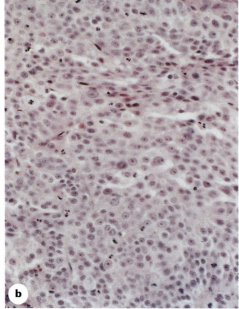

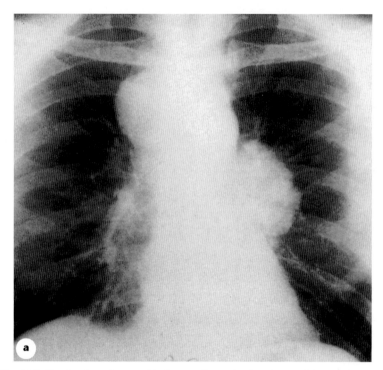

Fig. 3.12 Small cell carcinoma. (a) Chest radiograph of a 46-year-old man who presented with a cough and chest pain shows bilateral mediastinal nodal metastases. Bronchoscopy was positive for small cell lung cancer. Combination chemotherapy and mediastinal irradiation resulted in complete remission.

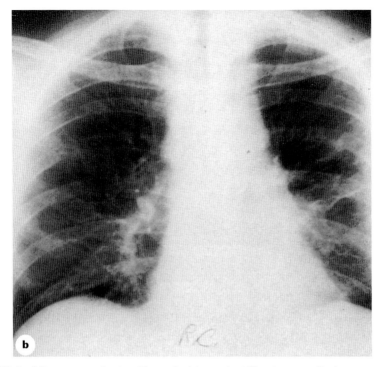

(b) On follow-up examination 18 months later, a chest film shows continuing remission.

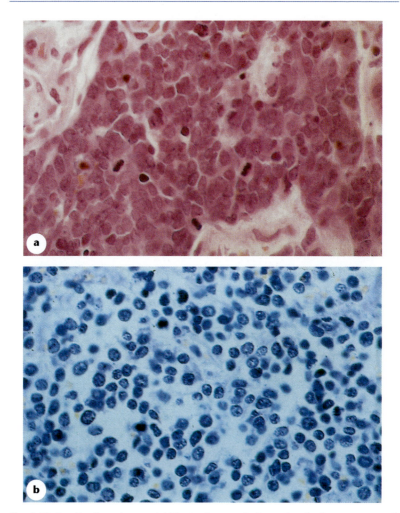

Fig. 3.13 Small cell carcinoma. (**a**) Photomicrograph shows the classic appearance of 'oat-like' cells. Each cell is approximately twice the size of a lymphocyte and has scant cytoplasm, finely dispersed chromatin and an inconspicuous nucleolus. Note characteristic 'molding' of the cells and a high mitotic rate. (**b**) In another case, the cells have a 'lymphocyte-like' appearance. Such tumours are included in the category of small cell lung cancer. Other malignancies that have a 'small cell' appearance include lymphomas, Merkel cell tumour, carcinoid tumours, rhabdomyosarcoma, Ewing's sarcoma and neuroblastoma.

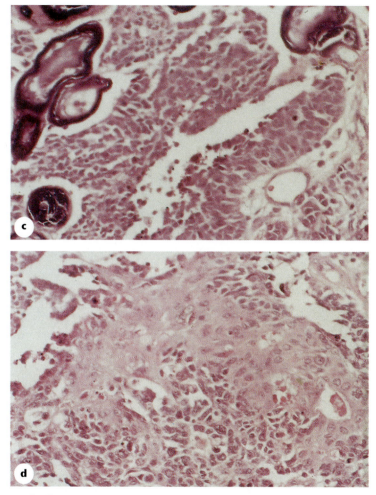

(c) Small cell carcinoma. This low-power view shows the Azzopardi effect, due to crushed DNA material encrusted around blood vessels, which is characteristic although not pathognomic of small cell carcinoma. (d) Small cell carcinoma, combined cell subtype. This tumour shows small cell and squamous cell components.

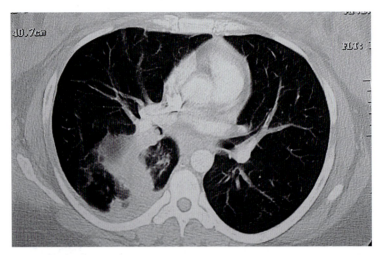

Fig. 3.14 Carcinoid tumour. Computed tomography scan shows an endobronchial mass filling the bronchus intermedius of this 24-year-old woman with a history of recurrent asthma and episodes of pneumonia. Note large area of consolidation due to the obstructing lesion.

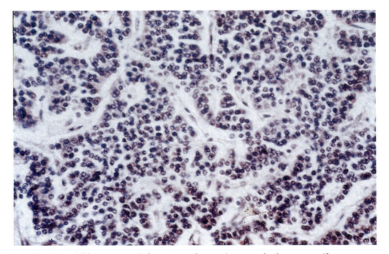

Fig. 3.15 Carcinoid tumour. High-power photomicrograph shows a uniform population of small, bland 'blue' cells with delicate nuclear chromatin and small amounts of cytoplasm. Note the organized arrangement of the tumour cells.

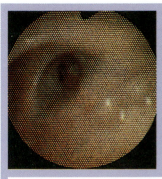

Fig. 3.16 T1N0 (stage IA) squamous cell carcinoma. Fibreoptic bronchoscopy reveals a 2 mm diameter lesion in the posterior segment of the right upper lobe bronchus.

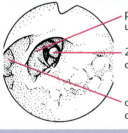

posterior segment of right upper lobe bronchus

2 mm diameter squamous cell carcinoma

orifice of apical segment of right upper lobe

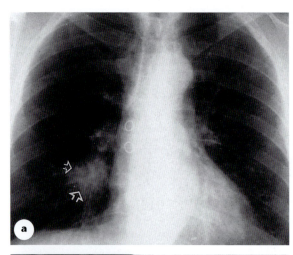

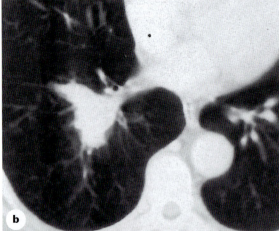

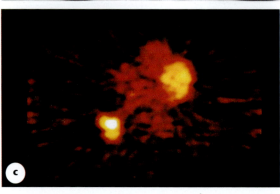

Fig. 3.17 T1N0 (stage IA) adenocarcinoma. (**a**) Posteroanterior chest film in a 60-year-old man with haemoptysis demonstrates a poorly defined, spiculated 2.5 cm mass in the right lower lobe (RLL) (arrows). The patient had a prior sternotomy and coronary artery bypass graft (CABG). (**b**) Computed tomography confirms the radiographically indeterminate RLL mass. (**c**) Axial position emission tomography image at the level of the mass demonstrates significantly increased uptake within the tumour, which was proven to be an adenocarcinoma by bronchoscopy. Note the normal increased activity in the left ventricle myocardium. Staging studies showed no metastases and a successful lobectomy was carried out. (Courtesy of Dr EF Patz Jr.)

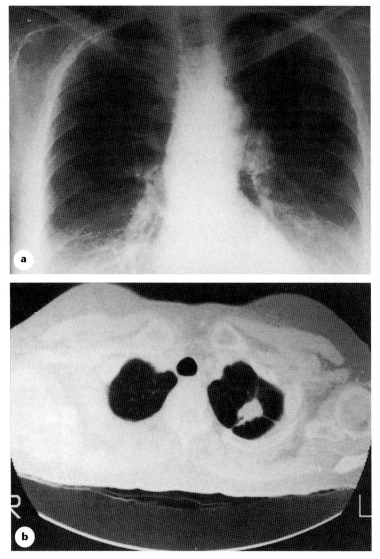

Fig. 3.18 T1N1 (stage IIA) poorly differentiated adenocarcinoma. This 56-year-old woman presented with recent onset of cough. (**a**) Chest radiograph shows left hilar adenopathy and a small lesion in the left upper lobe. Computed tomography scans confirm (**b**) a 1.5–2.0 cm primary lesion in the left upper lobe and

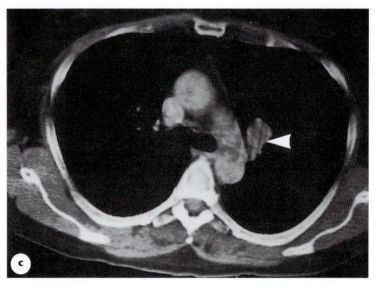

Fig. 3.18 *Continued* (c) an enlarged left hilar node (arrow). No mediastinal adenopathy was present and the tumour was successfully resected.

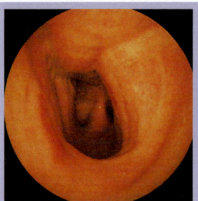

Fig. 3.19 T3N0 (stage IIA) lung cancer. Bronchoscopy demonstrates extrinsic compression of the left lower trachea and distortion of the carina and right bronchus by tumour. The cancer was within 2 cm of the carina but without invasion of the carina or trachea. This image was made via a rigid bronchoscope for clarity; it is oriented for a bronchoscopist standing in front of the subject. (Courtesy of Dr P Stradling.)

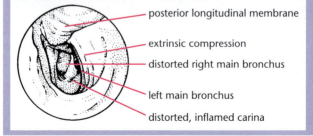

posterior longitudinal membrane

extrinsic compression

distorted right main bronchus

left main bronchus

distorted, inflamed carina

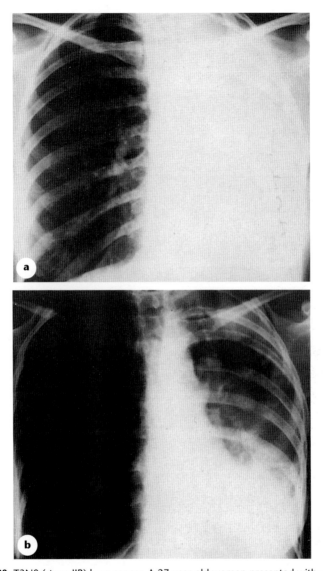

Fig. 3.20 T3N0 (stage IIB) lung cancer. A 27-year-old woman presented with increasing cough and sudden shortness of breath. (**a**) Chest radiograph shows complete collapse of the left lung. At bronchoscopy, a tumour was identified at the orifice of the left main bronchus. (**b**) Chest film following treatment shows re-expansion of the upper lobe. Involvement of the proximal bronchus within 2 cm of the carina, but not involvement of the carina itself, constitutes T3N0 (stage IIB) disease that is marginally resectable.

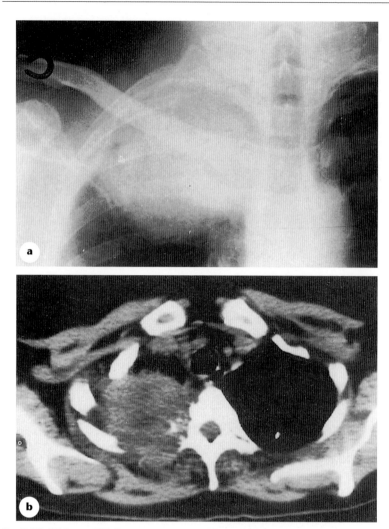

Fig. 3.21 T4 (stage IIIB) Pancoast tumour. A 52-year-old woman presented with long-standing right shoulder and back pain. (**a**) Her chest film shows a large tumour of the right upper lobe that has destroyed the adjacent rib. (**b**) Computed tomography scan reveals rib and soft tissue involvement as well as destruction of an adjacent vertebral body. Biopsy showed a squamous cell carcinoma. While in the past Pancoast (superior sulcus) tumours were mostly squamous cell carcinomas, many centres are now reporting more adenocarcinomas than squamous cell type, similar to other lung cancers. Large cell carcinoma is third in frequency while small cell carcinoma rarely presents as a Pancoast tumour.

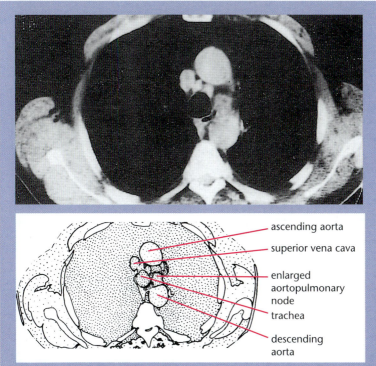

Fig. 3.22 N2 (stage IIIA) adenocarcinoma. A 47-year-old man with a primary tumour of the left upper lobe presented with hoarseness. Indirect laryngoscopy showed paralysis of the left vocal cord. This computed tomography scan reveals an enlarged lymph node in the aortopulmonary window, which was not seen on chest radiography. Anterior mediastinotomy (Chamberlain procedure) confirmed a metastatic tumour in the mediastinal node that compressed the recurrent laryngeal nerve, resulting in hoarseness.

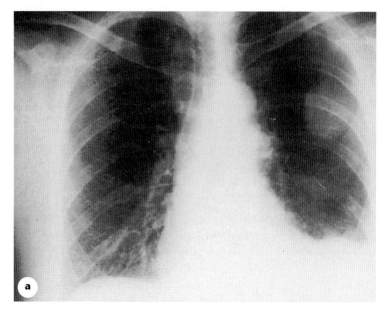

Fig. 3.23 T4 (stage IIIB) adenocarcinoma. A 61-year-old woman developed increasing left chest wall pain with dyspnoea on exertion. (a) Chest radiograph shows a pleural-based tumour mass with a pleural effusion.

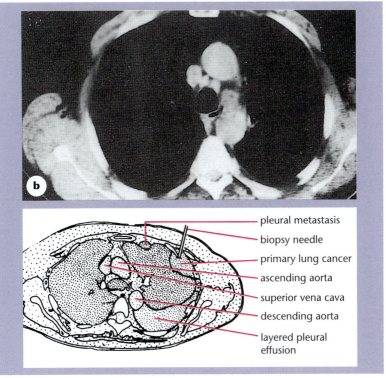

(**b**) Computed tomography (CT) scan confirms these findings and reveals a second small pleural metastasis. CT-guided needle biopsy showed a non-small cell lung cancer; thoracocentesis was positive for a poorly differentiated adenocarcinoma. Mammograms and other staging studies were normal.

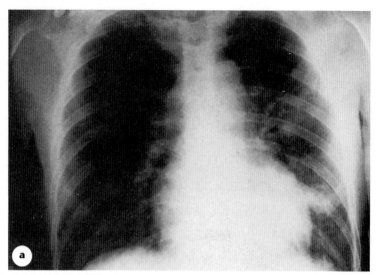

Fig. 3.24 T4 (stage IIIB) adenocarcinoma. A 62-year-old woman presented with severe dyspnoea at rest. (**a**) Chest film shows a tumour mass in the left lower lobe associated with cardiomegaly due to pericardial effusion with acute tamponade, findings that are confirmed on computed tomography scan (**b**). Histopathological specimens obtained by pericardiocentesis showed poorly differentiated adenocarcinoma cells that were positive for cytokeratin 7 and thyroid transcription factor-1 but negative for cytokeratin 20, consistent with lung cancer.[13] Radiotherapy was administered. (**c**) Follow-up chest film reveals an improvement in heart size but persistence of the primary tumour mass. A vascular access device has also been placed.

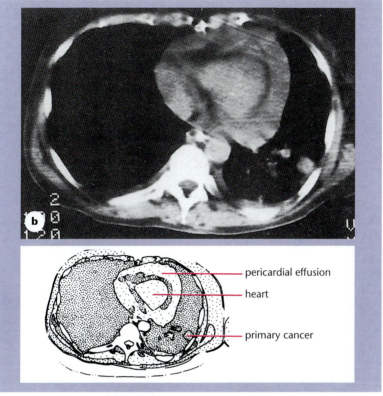

pericardial effusion

heart

primary cancer

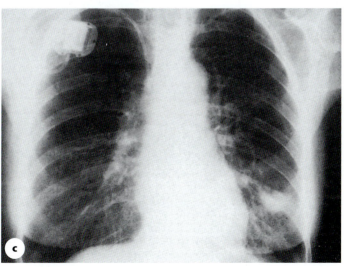

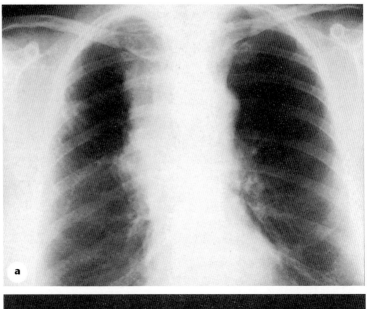

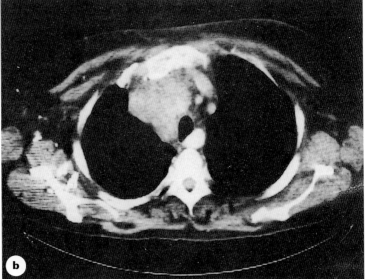

Fig. 3.25 T4 (stage IIIB) squamous cell carcinoma (superior vena cava syndrome). A 45-year-old woman developed increasing facial oedema, distended neck veins, enlarged breasts and shortness of breath. (a) Chest radiograph reveals a large mass in the right upper lung and mediastinum. (b) Computed tomography scan shows encasement of the superior vena cava by the primary tumour mass.

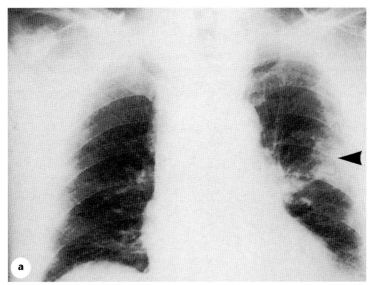

Fig. 3.26 N3 (stage IIIB) poorly differentiated adenocarcinoma. A 67-year-old man complained of increasing cough, chest discomfort and weight loss. (a) Chest radiograph shows a lesion (arrow) in the left upper lobe.

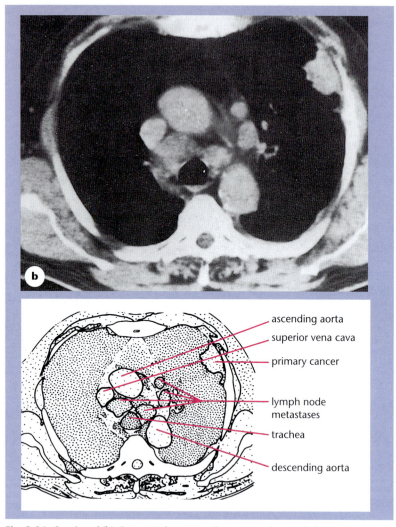

Fig. 3.26 *Continued* (**b**) Computed tomography scan confirms a 2–3 cm primary lung tumour (T2) based in the pleura and reveals in addition bilateral mediastinal lymph node metastases. Bronchoscopy was negative, but needle biopsy of the primary lesion yielded the histological diagnosis.

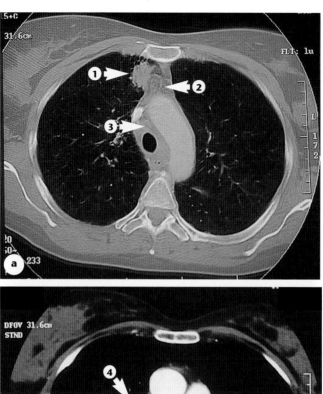

Fig. 3.27 T1N3 (stage IIIB) adenocarcinoma of the lung. A 44-year-old woman presented with an enlarged supraclavicular lymph node mass. Biopsy showed metastatic adenocarcinoma that was positive for thyroid transcription factor-1 and cytokeratin 7 but negative for cytokeratin 20, consistent with lung cancer. At age 18, she was treated for stage IIIB Hodgkin's disease with MOPP chemotherapy followed by mantle field irradiation. Prior therapy, especially radiotherapy, leads to a higher incidence of second primary malignancies such as lung cancer. Computed tomography scan shows: (**a**) the primary cancer in the medial right upper lobe (1), left (2) and right (3) mediastinal nodes; (**b**) right hilar (4) and subcarinal (5) nodes.

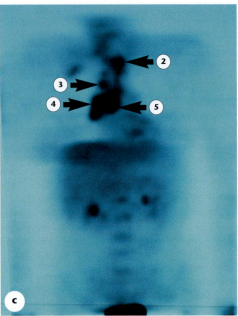

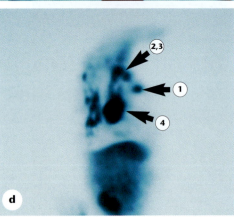

Fig. 3.27 *Continued* A staging position emission tomography (PET) scan reveals: (**c**) coronal image: right hilar (4), subcarinal (5) and upper mediastinal (2,3) nodes; (**d**) sagittal image: primary cancer (1), upper mediastinal (2,3) and right hilar (4) nodes. Normal liver uptake and renal excretion are noted. No other metastases were evident. The diagnostic role of thyroid transcription factor-1 is discussed by Ordonez[7] while the value of PET staging is reviewed by Pieterman *et al.*[14] (Courtesy of Milos Janicek MD, PhD, Department of Radiology, Brigham and Women's Hospital and Dana-Farber Cancer Institute, Boston, MA.)

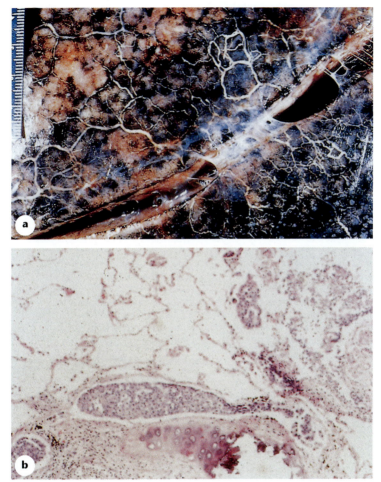

Fig. 3.28 Pulmonary lymphangitis carcinomatosa. (**a**) The pleural surface of this autopsy specimen from a patient who died of a poorly differentiated non-small cell lung cancer shows dilated lymphatic channels filled with tumour. (**b**) Microscopic section of the lung demonstrates malignant cells infiltrating lymphatic channels.

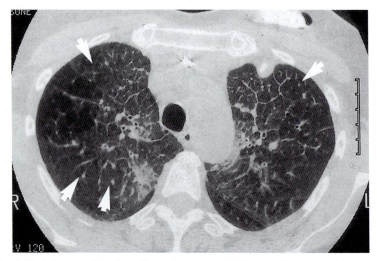

Fig. 3.29 Pulmonary lymphangitis carcinomatosa. A 49-year-old woman with previous resection of a poorly differentiated adenocarcinoma of the lung presented with increasing dyspnoea on exertion. Chest radiograph showed non-diagnostic features. Computed tomography image at the level of the aortic arch displayed with lung windows shows bilateral thickening of interlobular septae consistent with lymphangitic tumour spread. The thickened septae (arrows) form polygons containing a central dot, representing a pulmonary vein.

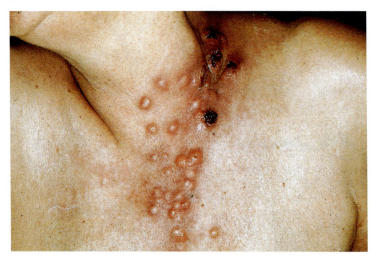

Fig. 3.30 Cutaneous metastases. A 48-year-old woman with a small cell lung cancer developed numerous skin lesions. Generalized skin or subcutaneous metastases, which may be quite painful, often occur and may be seen in all histological subtypes. In some patients, a solitary early skin metastasis may be the presenting sign of an underlying lung tumour.

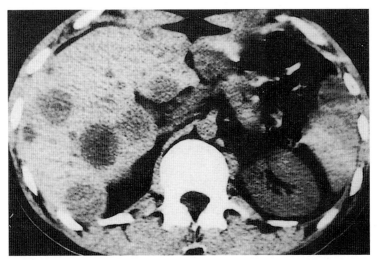

Fig. 3.31 Liver metastases. Computed tomography (CT) scan of a 28-year-old man with metastatic atypical carcinoid tumour shows numerous metastatic liver deposits which developed after control of his primary pulmonary malignancy by surgery. CT is quite accurate in detecting early metastases and use of contrast with CT helps rule out benign cysts, which do not enhance with contrast. Ultrasound can also differentiate cystic from solid lesions. These lesions would also be evident by magnetic resonance imaging and position emission tomography.

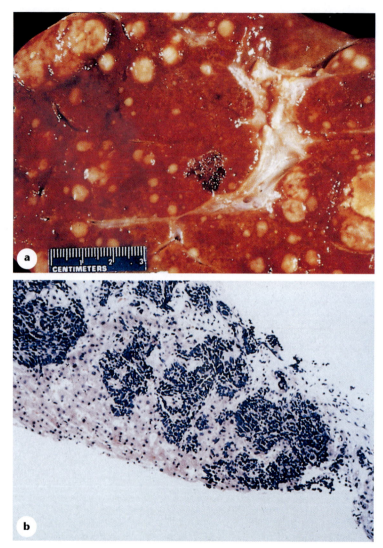

Fig. 3.32 Liver metastases. (**a**) Autopsy specimen from a patient who died of widespread small cell lung cancer exhibits numerous lesions ranging in size from a few millimeters to 1–2 cm. A similar pattern can be seen with non-small cell carcinomas. (**b**) Photomicrograph of a liver biopsy from a patient with small cell lung tumour shows marked involvement by clumps of undifferentiated dark-staining cells.

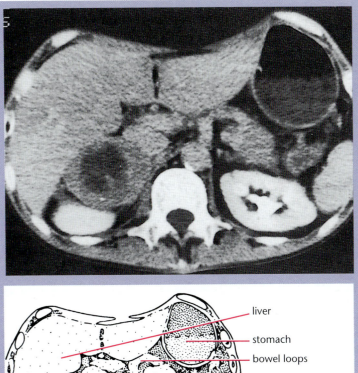

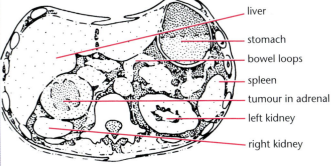

liver

stomach

bowel loops

spleen

tumour in adrenal

left kidney

right kidney

Fig. 3.33 Adrenal metastases. Abdominal computed tomography scan of a patient with a non-small cell lung cancer shows a large metastatic lesion in the right adrenal gland; central tumour necrosis is also evident. This patient was considered for surgery before the adrenal lesion was detected. About 5–10% of patients with localized lung cancer on chest radiography have asymptomatic adrenal metastases. Carcinoma of the lung is by far the most common source of adrenal metastases, followed by carcinoma of the breast and malignant melanoma. In general, adrenal metastases are bilateral and most often appear first in the medulla. Cortical involvement is also common and in rare cases such metastatic spread may give rise to Addison's disease.

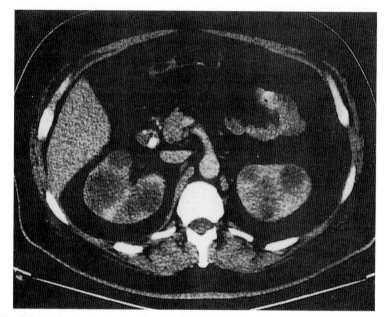

Fig. 3.34 Kidney metastases. Computed tomography scan shows bilateral renal metastases in a 63-year-old man who also had liver and bone involvement by a primary adenocarcinoma of the lung. Renal cysts can usually be ruled out by ultrasound.

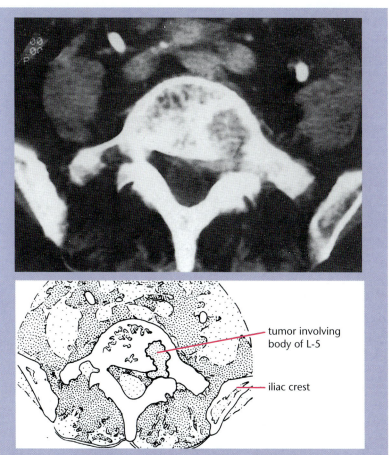

tumor involving
body of L-5

iliac crest

Fig. 3.35 Bone metastases. A 74-year-old woman presented with pain and weakness of the left leg. A right lower lobe mass was noted on her chest radiograph and a diagnosis of adenocarcinoma was subsequently made by bronchoscopy. Computed tomography scan shows compression of the cauda equina by tumour involving the body of L5. Her leg pain and weakness dramatically improved after radiotherapy.

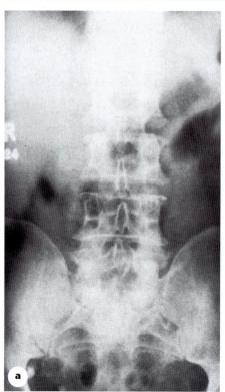

Fig. 3.36 Bone metastases. (**a**) Radiograph of the lumbar spine in a patient who had a bronchial carcinoma and complained of back pain indicates no abnormality. However, radionuclide bone scans (**b, c**) reveal multiple metastases in the lumbar spine and pelvis, as well as deposits in the thoracic vertebrae and ribs.

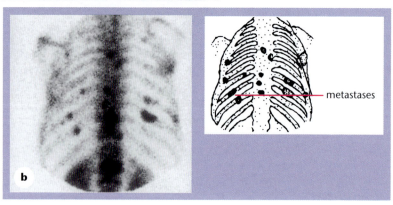

metastases

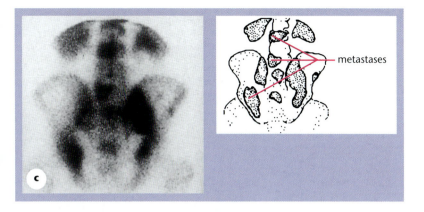

metastases

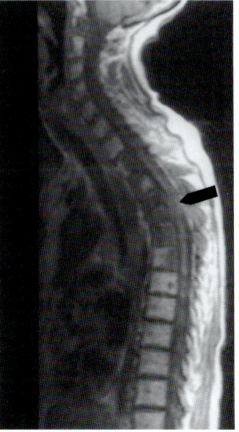

Fig. 3.37 Bone marrow metastases. A 62-year-old woman presented with upper back pain and neurological findings diagnostic of early spinal cord compression. Normal bone marrow appears white on this T2-weighted magnetic resonance imaging scan due to fat content, except in the upper spine where metastatic lung cancer has replaced the bone marrow and appears black. The spinal cord appears white and shows an area of displacement due to compression by tumour invading through the intervertebral space (arrow).

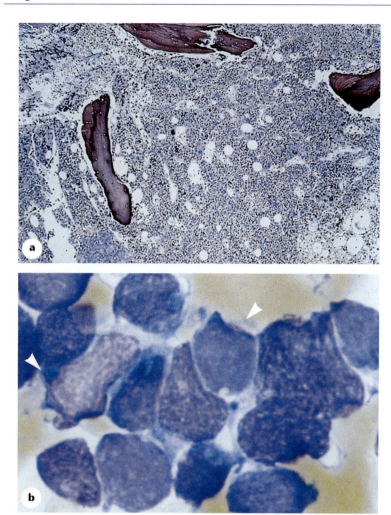

Fig. 3.38 Bone marrow metastases. (**a**) Low-power photomicrograph of a bone marrow biopsy specimen shows focal involvement by metastatic small cell lung cancer. (**b**) High-power view of a bone marrow aspirate shows a cluster of malignant small cells with prominent nuclear molding (arrows). The differential diagnosis of this cytology includes other small blue cell malignancies, e.g. Ewing's sarcoma, neuroblastoma, rhabdomyosarcoma, and lymphoma. Bone marrow involvement as the only site of metastatic disease occurs in 5–10% of cases; the incidence rises to 40% or greater when metastases are found at other sites.

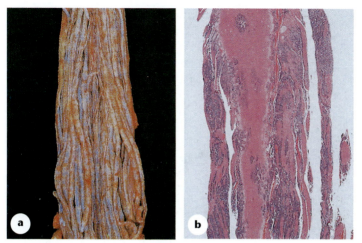

Fig. 3.39 Leptomeningeal metastases. (**a**) The red hypervascular patches on the nerve roots of the cauda equina in this fresh specimen represent leptomeningeal deposits of a metastatic lung carcinoma. The cauda equina is a favourite location for this process. (**b**) Whole-mount section of the specimen, which better demonstrates the extent of infiltration, shows ropy thickening of individual nerve roots by dense, blue-staining tumour cell nuclei. Minor extension of tumour into the spinal cord is also evident.

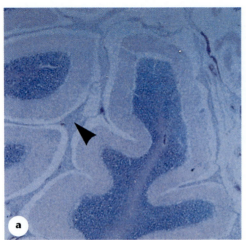

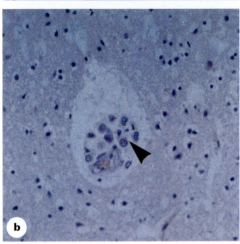

Fig. 3.40 Leptomeningeal metastases. A 55-year-old man was diagnosed with an undifferentiated large cell lung cancer. Two months later, he presented with headache followed by numbness of the hands. Examination showed diplopia, dysarthria, nystagmus, palsies of the left VI and right VII cranial nerves, bilateral limb ataxia, areflexia and gait ataxia. (**a**) Section of cerebellum shows infiltration of the leptomeninges by malignant cells (arrow) and, on high-power view (**b**), invasion of the Virchow–Robin space (arrow).

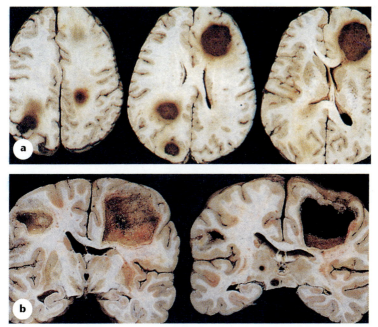

Fig. 3.41 Brain metastases. (**a**) Gross specimens show metastatic deposits of an undifferentiated large cell lung carcinoma. The metastases form essentially necrotic masses with peripheral enhancement and peritumoural oedema. (**b**) Occasionally, extensive necrosis transforms metastases into cysts lined by only a thin rim of viable tumour.

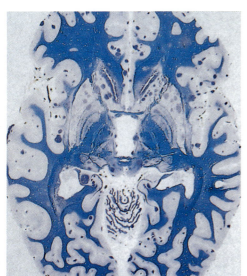

Fig. 3.42 Brain metastases. Horizontal whole-mount section of a brain shows metastatic small cell lung carcinoma as miliary cerebral metastases. Many are situated in grey matter or at the grey–white matter junction. The ventricular surface is also involved. Note the relative sparing of white matter and the absence of oedema.

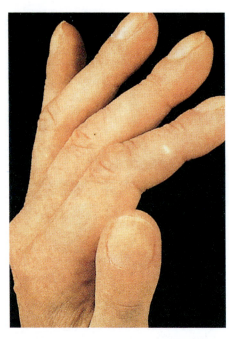

Fig. 3.43 Hypertrophic pulmonary osteoarthropathy (HPO). A characteristic manifestation of HPO, digit clubbing occurs in about 10% of lung cancer patients of all histological subgroups, but particularly in adenocarcinoma. The disease may be early or advanced. Benign tumours, inflammatory disease and liver disease are also associated with clubbing. While the pathophysiology is poorly understood, digital clubbing, painful joints and tender extremities – features commonly seen in HPO – often reverse dramatically after successful thoracotomy, radiotherapy or chemotherapy.

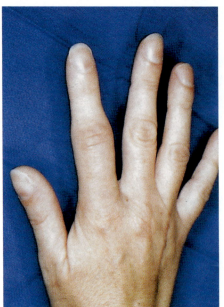

Fig. 3.44 HPO and digital metastases. This 45-year-old woman presented with HPO and also pain and swelling of her right index finger. Radiographs showed lytic lesions in the middle phalanx and bone scan was positive in this area (not shown). Biopsy was positive for metastatic, poorly differentiated adenocarcinoma from the lung. Metastases to bone beyond the humerus and/or femur are unusual in any type of primary cancer.

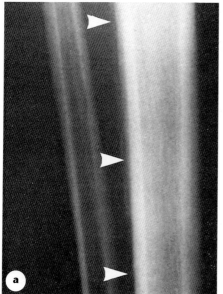

Fig. 3.45 Hypertrophic pulmonary osteoarthropathy (periostitis). (a) Radiograph of the lower leg shows periosteal elevation (arrows) in the tibia of a patient who presented with joint pain of the lower legs and feet. Evaluation subsequently showed a primary lung adenocarcinoma of the right upper lobe (b, c) Bone scans show focal increased uptake of radiopharmaceutical in both legs in areas of new bone formation; no bone metastases are evident.

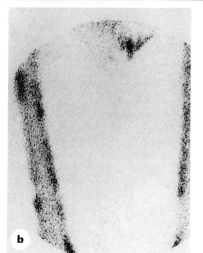

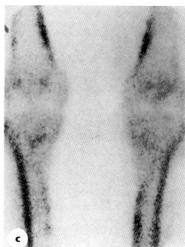

Table 3.2 Lesions causing a mass on chest radiography

Neoplastic	Infective	Miscellaneous
Malignant	Bacterial	Sarcoidosis
Primary lung carcinoma	Viral	Rheumatoid nodules
Carcinoid tumour	Lung abscess	Pseudolymphoma
Lymphoma	Empyema	Wegener's granulomatosis
Plasmacytoma		Bronchocentric granulomatosis
Thymoma	Tuberculosis	Echinococcal cyst
Germ cell tumour	Tuberculoma	Pseudotumour (fluid)
Sarcoma		
Metastatic carcinoma	Fungal	Amyloidosis
	Aspergilloma	Castleman's disease
Benign	Allergic aspergillosis	
Neurofibroma	Histoplasmoma	
Hamartoma	Mycetoma	
Pulmonary embolism		
Thyroid goitre	Parasite	
Cyst		
Arteriovenous malformation		

Table 3.3 Diagnostic methods for assessment of mass lesions

Fibreoptic bronchoscopy	Radiology	Transthoracic biopsy*
Bronchial tree secretions, bacteriology and cytology	Plain PA and lateral views	Fine needle aspiration
	Computed tomography (CT)	Cutting needle biopsy
Bronchial biopsy	Magnetic resonance imaging (MRI)	Video assisted thoracoscopic biopsy/resection
Transbronchial biopsy		
Transbronchial needle aspiration		
Thoracotomy	PET scanning	
	Angiography (not often used)	
Selective bronchial brushing		
Bronchioalveolar lavage		

*When the biopsy studies given here are negative, mediastinoscopy or mediastinotomy may be indicated in selected patients

Table 3.4 Causes of interstitial lung abnormalities

The finding of an interstitial pattern on chest radiography may be the result of numerous causes, among them lung neoplasia

Neoplastic	Immunological	Occupational	Infectious	Drug-related	Rare
Multiple metastatic tumours, primary or secondary	Collagen-vascular diseases	Asbestosis Silicosis	Miliary tuberculosis Fungal infection (e.g. candidiasis)	Amiodarone Cytotoxic drugs Paraquat	Haemosiderosis Eosinophilic granuloma
Bronchioloalveolar carcinoma	Cryptogenic fibrosing alveolitis	Siderosis	Protozoan infection (e.g. pneumocystis)		Alveolar proteinosis
Lymphangitis carcinomatosa	Extrinsic allergic alveolitis	Talcosis	Viral infection (e.g. cytomegalovirus)		
Leukaemia	Pulmonary eosinophilia				
Lymphoma	Granulomatous disorders				

Table 3.5 Manifestations of selected paraneoplastic syndromes in lung cancer patients by type of manifestation and frequency[4]

Type of manifestation	Frequency (%)
Systemic	
Anorexia-cachexia	31
Fever	21
Suppressed immunity	
Skeletal	
Digital clubbing	29
Periostitis (hypertrophic pulmonary osteoarthropathy) – commonly associated with adenocarcinoma	1–10
Endocrine	
Hypercalcaemia (ectopic parathyroid hormone) – commonly associated with squamous cell carcinoma	
Hyponatraemia (inappropriate secretion of ADH) – commonly associated with small cell carcinoma	
Cushing's syndrome (ectopic ACTH secretion) – commonly associated with small cell carcinoma	
Haematologic	8
Anaemia	
Granulocytosis	
Eosinophilia	
Leukoerythroblastosis	
Coagulation – thrombotic	1–4
Venous thrombosis (migratory thrombophlebitis, Trousseau's syndrome)	
Arterial embolism (non-bacterial thrombotic endocarditis)	
Haemorrhage (disseminated Intravascular coagulation)	
Neurologic – myopathic	1
Eaton–Lambert syndrome (myasthenia) – commonly associated with small cell carcinoma	
Peripheral neuropathy	
Subacute cerebellar degeneration	
Cortical degeneration	
Polymyositis	
Neurologic – cutaneous	1
Dermatomyositis	
Acanthosis nigricans	
Renal	< 1
Nephrotic syndrome	
Glomerulonephritis	

ADH, antidiuretic hormone; ACTH, adrenocorticotropic hormone

REFERENCES

1. Devesa SS, Bray F, Vizcaino AP, Parkin DM: International lung cancer trends by histologic type: male:female differences diminishing and adenocarcinoma rates rising. Int J Cancer 2005; 117(2): 294–299.
2. Jemal A, Siegel R, Ward E, et al: Cancer statistics, 2007. CA Cancer J Clin 2007; 57: 43–66.
3. Doll R, Peto R, Boreham J, Sutherland I: Mortality in relation to smoking: 50 years' observations on male doctors. BMJ 2004; 328 (7445): 1519.
4. Minna JD, Pass H, Glatstein EJ: Cancer of the lung. In: DeVita VT Jr. Hellman S, Rosenberg SA, eds: Cancer: principles and practice of oncology, 3rd edn. Lippincott, Philadelphia, 1989: 591–724.
5. Travis WD, Colby TV, Corrin B, et al: Histological typing of lung and pleural tumors, 3rd edn. Springer Verlag, Berlin, 1999.
6. Alberg AJ, Brock MV, Samet JM: Epidemiology of lung cancer: looking to the future. J Clin Oncol 2005; 23(14): 3175–3185.
7. Ordonez NG: Value of thyroid transcription factor-1, E-cadherin, BG8, WT1, and CD44S immunostaining in distinguishing epithelial pleural mesothelioma from pulmonary and nonpulmonary adenocarcinoma. Am J Surg Pathol 2000; 24: 598–606.
8. Miller VA, Hirsch FR, Johnson DH: Systemic therapy of advanced bronchioloalveolar cell carcinoma: challenges and opportunities. J Clin Oncol 2005; 23(14): 3288–3293.
9. Travis WD, Brambilla E, et al: Pathology and genetics of tumours of the lung, pleura, thymus and heart. World Health Organization Classification of Tumours, 2004. Ed. Travis WD. IARC Press, Lyon.
10. Gadzar, AF, et al: Molecular targets for cancer therapy and prevention. CHEST 2004; 125:97S–101S.
11. Lynch TJ, Bell DW, Sordella R, et al: Activating mutations in the epidermal growth factor receptor: underlying responsiveness of non-small-cell lung cancer to gefitinib. N Engl J Med 2004; 350(21): 2129–2139.
12. Paez JG, Janne PA, Lee JC, et al: EGFR mutations in lung cancer: correlation with clinical response to gefitinib therapy. Science 2004; 304: 1497–1500.
13. Rubin BP, Skarin AT, Pisick E, et al: Use of cytokeratins 7 and 20 in determining the origin of metastatic carcinoma of unknown primary, with special emphasis on lung cancer. Eur J Cancer Prev 2001; 10: 77–82.
14. Pieterman RM, van Putten JWG, Meuzelaar JJ, et al: Preoperative staging of non-small cell lung cancer with positron-emission tomography. N Engl J Med 2000; 343: 254–261.

FIGURE CREDITS

The following books published by Gower Medical Publishing are sources of figures in the present chapter. The figure numbers given in the listing are those of the figures in the present chapter. The page numbers (or slide numbers) given in parentheses are those of the original publication.
Dieppe PA, Bacon PA, Bamji AN, et al.: Atlas of clinical rheumatology. Lea & Febiger/Gower Medical Publishing, Philadelphia/London, 1986: Fig 3.36 (p 21.6), Table 3.5 (p 21.2).

du Bois RM, Clarke SW: Fibreoptic bronchoscopy in diagnosis and management. Lippincott/Gower Medical Publishing, Philadelphia/London, 1987: Table 3.2 (p 3.2), Table 3.3 (p 3.2), Table 3.4 (p 4.2), 3.16 (p 3.8), 3.19 (p 3.11), 3.20 (p 6.18).

Okazaki H, Scheithauer BW: Atlas of neuropathology. Lippincott/Gower Medical Publishing, Philadelphia/New York, 1988: Figs 3.39 (p 168), 3.41 (p 171), 3.42 (p 170).

Perkin GD, Rose FC, Blackwood W, et al.: Atlas of clinical urology. Lippincott/Gower Medical Publishing, Philadelphia/London, 1986: Fig 3.40 (p 9.8).

Spencer H, ed: Respiratory system. In: Turk JL, Fletcher CDM, eds: RCSE slide atlas of pathology. Gower Medical Publishing, London, 1986: Figs 3.2 (slide 68), 3.4 (slide 91).

Lung cancer: screening, staging and treatment

Arthur T. Skarin and Christopher Lathan

SCREENING

Given the high incidence and mortality of lung cancer in industrialized countries, and the fact that so many patients present with advanced disease, the search for a screening technique that might decrease mortality by detecting earlier stage disease seems appropriate. Original studies conducted in the 1970s that examined sputum analysis and chest radiography as screening modalities in current and former smokers found no evidence that sputum analysis or annual chest X-rays decreased lung cancer mortality. Chest X-rays were not deemed sensitive enough to pick up lesions <2 cm.[1]

Screening studies were revived in the 1990s using spiral computer-assisted tomography (CT) scans. Single-institution studies confirmed that screening with spiral CT scans increased the number of early stage lung cancers detected; however many patients were found to have benign non-calcified lesions, and as such the cost-effectiveness of screening current and former smokers with spiral CT scan has been debated.[2]

At present there are no randomized data available to show a benefit for CT screening and there is no recommended screening strategy for non-small cell lung cancer (NSCLC). The International Early Lung Trialists Action Programme (I-ELCAP) recently reported on 31,567 asymptomatic persons at risk of lung cancer screened from 1993 through 2005. Eighty-five percent of the cancers detected were stage I; the estimated 10-year survival of those with stage I disease was 88%, higher than the generally reported range of 70% for these patients. The ongoing National Cancer Institute (NCI) sponsored National Lung Cancer Screening Trial is a randomized study that allocates subjects to either chest X-ray or CT screening. Accrual of 50,000 patients was completed in 2004 and first results are expected in 2009. This randomized trial will provide information about mortality reduction and cost-effectiveness of screening.

STAGING OF NSCLC

The most widely used system is the International Staging System (ISS) using TNM categories to place patients into stages I–IV, each having a progressively poorer survival rate (see Figure 4.1). It was revised in 1997 with additional stage subgroupings (see also Figure 4.2).[3] Approximately 30% of patients present with stage I or II disease; 15–20% have potentially resectable stage IIIA disease and the remainder have advanced unresectable stage IIIB or metastatic stage IV disease. Given that stage determines survival and type of treatment, the accurate staging of NSCLC is of the utmost importance.[4]

Staging procedures consist of a CT scan of the chest and upper abdomen to include the liver and adrenals. Other investigations include isotope bone scan, brain scan, tumour markers etc., and should be performed based on local/national guidelines and/or clinical suspicion. The recent guidelines from the American Society of Clinical Oncology on treatment of NSCLC include advice on staging of patients, and these are broadly set out below.[5]

LYMPH NODE STATUS

Accurate evaluation of mediastinal lymph nodes is the key to accurate staging.[6,7] Invasive staging procedures include bronchoscopy, thoracoscopy, cervical (suprasternal) mediastinoscopy and anterior mediastinoscopy (Chamberlain procedure). One or more may be carried out to evaluate mediastinal nodal stations (see Figure 4.3) or suspicious sites of disease in resectable patients, particularly when multimodality treatment protocols are utilized. Video-assisted thoracoscopic surgery is often utilized for staging as well as treatment in selected cases (see Figure 4.4). The technique has minimal mortality and greatly reduces hospitalization time compared with traditional thoracotomy.[6,8] Endoscopic bronchoscopic ultrasound is increasingly being used for staging of potentially resectable tumours,[9] and endoscopic ultrasound–guided fine–needle aspiration is another invasive staging procedure that allows for biopsy of mediastinal lymph nodes. Although not used as extensively, this procedure is less invasive and costly than mediastinoscopy.[7,10]

POSITRON-EMISSION TOMOGRAPHY (PET)

The role of PET scans in the mediastinal staging of NSCLC has been evolving over the past decade, and PET/CT is now a core imaging

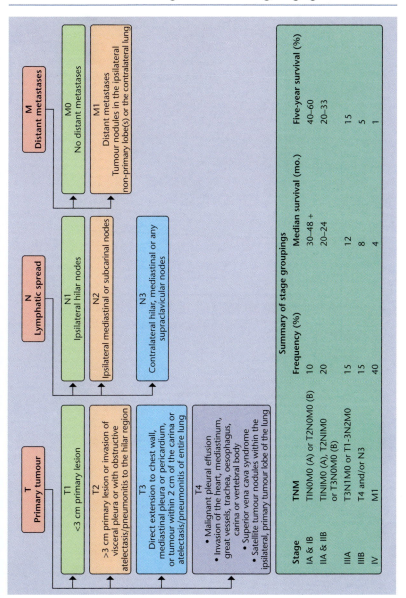

Fig. 4.1 International Staging System for lung cancer (simplified from Refs. 3 and 21). The frequency of each clinical stage varies, depending upon patient referral patterns. Survival is based upon clinical staging. Survival for surgically staged patients is higher in resected cases. Not indicated above: TX – malignant cells in bronchopulmonary secretions but primary cancer not otherwise visualized; T0 – no evidence of primary tumour; Tis – carcinoma *in situ*.

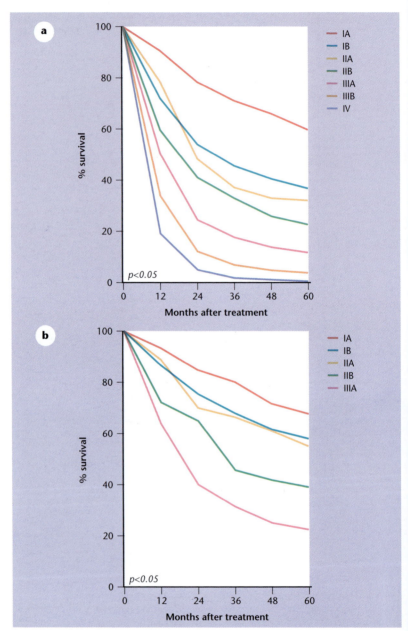

Fig. 4.2 A cumulative proportion of patients expected to survive following treatment according to (**a**) clinical estimates of the stage of disease and (**b**) surgical-pathological stage.[3]

technique for staging potentially resectable tumours. Whole-body PET using ^{18}F-fluorodeoxyglucose as a tracer is an imaging technique based upon the increased metabolism of glucose in malignant cells. PET has a 95% sensitivity for detecting primary lung cancers and mediastinal lymph node involvement.[11,12] It has not replaced invasive biopsy of the mediastinum but can be used to provide more information during the staging process.[7,11–17] The threshold of detection is around 3–5 mm. It

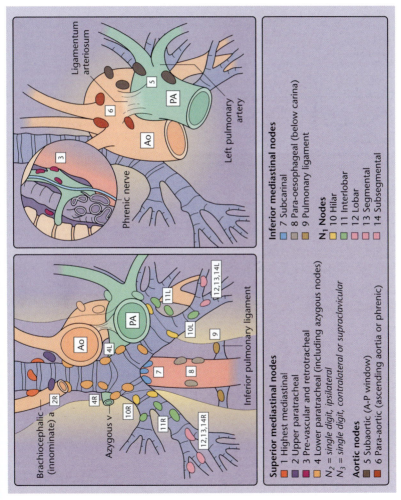

Fig. 4.3 Regional nodal stations for lung cancer staging.[3]

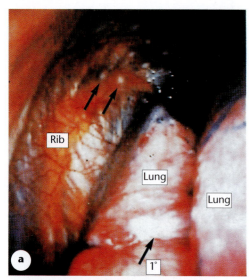

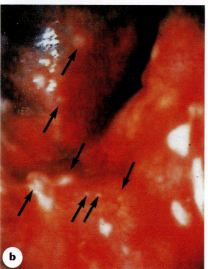

Fig. 4.4 T4 (stage IIIB) adenocarcinoma. A 44-year-old woman presented with increasing cough and the chest radiograph (not shown) revealed a 2 cm infiltrative lesion in the left lower lobe (**a**, 1° tumour). Computed tomography scan showed no mediastinal adenopathy but some small pleural densities were present (not shown). VATS (video-assisted thoracoscopic surgery) was carried out and revealed multiple small visceral and parietal pleural nodules (arrows, **b**). Biopsies were positive for metastatic adenocarcinoma unresectable stage IIIB disease. The patient was spared a formal thoracotomy by the staging VATS procedure.

may more accurately predict the likelihood of long-term survival than chest CT does.[18,19] Evaluation and restaging by PET/CT can also be very useful in assessing the response to induction therapy in patients with locally advanced disease, where repeat surgical staging may not be possible due to adhesions or fibrosis. PET is also useful to differentiate benign from malignant pulmonary nodules, assess response to treatment and recurrence, and assist in radiotherapy planning.[18] Bone metastases in NSCLC can be diagnosed with high accuracy by bone scans. At many centres, however, PET scanning has replaced bone scans since bone metastases, whether osteolytic, osteoblastic or mixed, will usually be detected by PET scans.

STAGING OF SMALL CELL LUNG CANCER

Although the ISS can be applied to all cell types, characterization of small cell lung cancer patients into limited and extensive stage disease has been the basis of treatment choice for a number of years. Patients are staged as limited or extensive stage disease based on the anatomical extent of the disease as proposed originally by the Veterans Administrator Lung Cancer Group and revised by the International Association for the Study of Lung Cancer.[20,21] Multivariate analysis studies have shown that a number of other factors have independent prognostic significance over and above anatomical staging. These include performance status and various biochemical factors. The Manchester Prognostic Score consists of five prognostic factors (tumour stage, performance status, serum sodium, alkaline phosphatase and serum lactate dehydrogenase).[22,23]

Using a cumulative risk score, patients fall into three main groups. Over 50% of patients with a prognostic score 0–1 will be alive at 1 year. Only 15% of patients with a score of 2–3 will be alive at 1 year; no patients with a score of 4–5 will be alive at 1 year. The identification of groups of patients with a better or worse prognosis has allowed the rational development of treatment approaches.

A number of other, similar prognostic scores have been devised, some including response to therapy.[24,25]

LUNG CANCER THERAPY

Appropriate treatment and therapeutic intent is determined by stage at presentation. Surgery is the primary therapy for stage I–II, if technically possible, but sadly only 20–30% of patients with lung cancer are suitable for resection. The appropriate treatment for stage III patients is an ongoing controversy in lung cancer management.[3] Given the possibility of cure in a proportion of patients, those with good performance status and pulmonary function should explore the curative option of multimodality therapy. The role of induction chemotherapy or combined chemoradiotherapy remains unclear and clinical trials are ongoing. Heterogeneity of patients and trial designs make it difficult to compare the outcomes of individual studies. At this time there is no consensus on induction chemotherapy or chemoradiotherapy, but appropriate management is best determined by a multidisciplinary team experienced in treating these patients.[26] Even when patients are surgical candidates, there are relatively high rates of both distant and local recurrences, with distant relapse predominating. This pattern of relapse suggests that some adjuvant treatment with chemotherapy might improve cure rates in lung cancer.

ADJUVANT RADIOTHERAPY IN NSCLC

Early enthusiasm for postoperative radiation in resected NSCLC was dimmed after the findings in the postoperative radiotherapy trial. The Radiation Therapy Oncology Group (RTOG) examined this question in 1998 with the publication of the controversial Post-Operative Radiotherapy (PORT) study. In this study, not only was postoperative radiation not helpful in prolonging life for most patients post-resection, but it was found to be detrimental to patients, most specifically resected patients with N0–1 disease.[27] Patients with N2 disease did not show evidence of the detrimental effect seen in the N0–1 group. Currently there is no role for postoperative radiation for stage I–II patients. Consideration of postoperative radiation when there is evidence of N2 or N3 disease is the subject of future studies. Controversy remains over the generalizability of the PORT study given that the study did not employ modern radiotherapy techniques.

ADJUVANT CHEMOTHERAPY IN NSCLC

Given the rate of distant metastasis in resected lung cancer, even definitive local therapy does not ensure the high survival rates that would be expected. The success of adjuvant treatment in breast and colon cancer has led many to explore this option in lung cancer. The addition of systemic chemotherapy postoperatively to patients to decrease distant metastasis in lung cancer has been tried in many forms. Although there were small single-institution studies that suggested an improvement in survival with chemotherapy, there were no definitive data to support adjuvant treatment until the meta-analysis by the Non-Small Cell Lung Cancer Collaborative Group. This study examined surgery alone vs. surgery followed by chemotherapy. Cisplatin-based chemotherapy given adjuvantly suggested a trend towards improving survival.[28] These studies prompted a wave of clinical trials to examine the role of cisplatin-based chemotherapy after surgery. In 2004, the International Adjuvant Lung Cancer Trial demonstrated a significant 4% overall improvement in survival for patients stage II–III treated adjuvantly with cisplatin-based chemotherapy.[29] Subsequent randomized clinical trials and two meta-analyses have supported this finding.[30–33] Results of five published recent randomized trials are summarized in Table 4.1.[34] Current recommendations are for stage II–III patients to consider

Table 4.1 Recent trials of adjuvant platinum-based chemotherapy in resected non-small cell lung cancer (NSCLC)

Study	Patients	Stage	Regimen	Hazard ratio	5-year survival (%)	P value
Scagliotti, et al.[64] ALPI 2003*	1209	I/II/IIIA	MVdP Observation	0.96	NR NR	0.589
Arriagada et al.[29] IALT 2004*	1867	I/II/III	P + E, Vd, Vn, or Vb Observation	0.86	44.5 40	<0.03
Strauss et al.[36] CALGB 2004	344	IB	TCp Observation	0.62	71+ 59+	0.028
Winton et al.[30] Intergroup 2005	482	IB/II	VnP Observation	0.69	69 54	0.04
Douillard et al.[31] ANITA 2005*	840	IB/II/IIIA	VnP Observation	0.79	51 43	0.013

*Allowed sequential radiation therapy according to oncologist preference
+4-year overall survival
ALPI, Adjuvant Lung Project Italy; ANITA, Adjuvant Navelbine International Trialists Association; CALGB, Cancer and Leukemia Group B; Cp, carboplatin; E, etoposide; I, ifosamide; IALT, International Adjuvant Lung Cancer Trialists; M, mitomycin C; NR, not reported; P, cisplatin; T, paclitaxel; Vb, vinblastine; Vd, vindesine; Vn, vinorelbine

adjuvant treatment with cisplatin and vinorelbine .[35] Studies are ongoing to determine the role of adjuvant treatment in stage IB disease, as well as determining if other platinum-based regimens are efficacious. Preliminary data presented in 2004 indicated that carboplatin/paclitaxel given IV every 21 days in a Cancer and Leukemia Group B (CALGB) sponsored study to patients who were postsurgery with stage IB NSCLC would benefit from adjuvant chemotherapy. The study was stopped early due to increased efficacy and led to many in the US adopting the carboplatin/paclitaxel regimen. Recent evaluation of mature data has called this into question and made the treatment of surgical stage IB NSCLC with carboplatin/paclitaxel an area of current study and controversy.[36] The role of adjuvant chemotherapy in stage IB disease remains unclear.

Studies from Japan using uracil-tegafur (UFT), an oral prodrug of fluorouracil, have shown a benefit for prolonged treatment with UFT for 2 years, or UFT + platinum chemotherapy for 1 year.[37] Studies in stage I and II disease also showed a benefit for single-agent UFT.[38,39] The applicability of these studies to a western population remains untested.

The role of newer agents including bevacizumab and epidermal growth factor receptor (EGFR) blocking drugs as adjuvant therapy is under evaluation.

The role of induction chemotherapy has been evaluated in four phase III trials. Three of the four studies had 60 patients or fewer; two showed a survival advantage. The results of a larger UK randomized trial are awaited.[40–43]

In summary, the role of neoadjuvant chemotherapy remains unproven but is promising. Studies comparing adjuvant with neoadjuvant chemotherapy are ongoing.

TREATMENT FOR LOCALLY ADVANCED NSCLC

Involvement of mediastinal lymph nodes drastically changes the likelihood of survival in NSCLC, with decreasing survival with N2 and N3 disease.[3,21] Over the past 16 years, the survival of this group has improved significantly with reported median survival in clinical trials increasing from 9.8 months to 17.7 months.

For patients with unresectable stage III disease, the role of chemotherapy and radiotherapy is somewhat clearer now. Three large studies in the 1990s showed a survival advantage for chemotherapy followed by radiotherapy, compared with radiotherapy alone.[44–46] The CALGB trial by Dillman et al was one of the first to show that combined radiation therapy and chemotherapy provided better survival than radiotherapy alone (13.7 months vs. 9.6 months).[44]

A number of studies then evaluated the role of concurrent chemoradiotherapy, exploiting the radiosensitizing effect of cisplatin. The majority showed a benefit for concurrent treatment.[47–51] The addition of maintenance/consolidation chemotherapy seemed to show a benefit in one study (Southwest Oncology Group; SWOG 9504);[52] this study is currently being evaluated in a phase III study by the Hoosier Oncology Group.

Two large phase III trials have examined the role of surgery after induction chemoradiotherapy. The Intergroup Study 0139 (RTOG 9309) examined patients with potentially resectable N2 disease. Patients received two cycles of fractionated cisplatin/etoposide with concurrent radiotherapy to 45 Gy. If there was no progression, patients were randomized to surgery or completion of radiotherapy to 61 Gy. Both groups then had two cycles of consolidation chemotherapy. Treatment-related mortality was significantly higher in the surgery arm, primarily in those treated with pneumonectomy, resulting in an early disadvantage for this arm. However, the overall survival curves crossed at 2 years with a trend towards improved overall survival at 5 years for trimodality therapy.[53] It is tempting to suggest that patients suitable for more limited surgery may benefit from this approach. A large randomized study from the German Lung Cancer Cooperative comparing chemotherapy followed by chemoradiotherapy followed by surgery, with chemotherapy followed by surgery followed by radiotherapy showed no difference in survival but increased toxicity for the chemoradiotherapy-treated patients.[54] This study had a number of design weaknesses and is difficult to interpret. The European Organisation for Research and Treatment of Cancer (EORTC) treated patients with stage IIIA (pN2) with three cycles of platinum-based chemotherapy. Responding patients were randomized between surgery (+/– postoperative radiotherapy) or radiotherapy alone. Three hundred and thirty-three patients were randomized. With a median follow-up of 6 years, there was no difference in outcome. An important feature of this study was the randomization of responding patients.[55]

When choosing the appropriate regimen for stage III lung cancer, clinical judgement and assessment of fitness determine which regimen should be used. Patients with borderline performance status should be considered for sequential treatment. Concurrent chemoradiotherapy remains the treatment of choice for fit patients with unresectable stage

III N2 disease; selected patients may benefit from limited surgery. The role of maintenance chemotherapy looks promising, but randomized data are awaited.

SUPERIOR SULCUS TUMOURS

The treatment of superior sulcus tumours, or Pancoast tumours, demonstrates the impact that multimodality therapy can make on a specific disease entity. Superior sulcus tumours usually arise in the apex of the lung, and were considered fatal until treatment with radiation and surgery was adopted. The majority of the primary tumours are T3–T4 by definition, and are usually stage IIB, IIIA or IIIB.[56] Patients should be thoroughly evaluated by a multimodality team, and imaging should include magnetic resonance imaging of the chest to evaluate the involvement of the brachial plexus.

Historical data indicate a poor outcome with surgery alone with a high risk of local recurrence, metastatic disease and postoperative complications. The addition of full-dose chemotherapy with radiation, followed by surgery, allowed for a more complete resection and improved outcomes dramatically.[26] Neoadjuvant chemotherapy and concurrent radiation became the standard of care in the SWOG Trial 9416. The current standard of care of superior sulcus tumours is induction with platinum-based chemoradiotherapy, followed by surgery. Resection rates after induction therapy were 92% with a 5-year survival of 41%.[56] For tumours that are not resectable, definitive chemotherapy and radiation should be given.

TREATMENT FOR STAGE IV NSCLC

The majority of patients with lung cancer have metastatic disease at presentation. Patients with either metastatic disease or a malignant pleural effusion have 5-year survival rates of 1–2%, and are not curable. The documentation of a malignant pleural effusion in a patient with locally advanced disease is often classified as a 'wet' IIIB. Prognosis and treatment for these patients is the same as stage IV.[3] The outcome of treatment is influenced by a number of prognostic factors, particularly performance status. Over the past 20 years, a treatment standard for advanced NSCLC has evolved for patients with good performance status. The goals of treatment in advanced NSCLC are palliation of symptoms and increasing survival. The argument for treatment of advanced NSCLC with chemotherapy was improved dramatically with the meta-analysis by the Non-Small Cell Lung Cancer Collaborative Group, which showed that cisplatin-based chemotherapy increased median survival by 1.5 months when compared with best supportive care.[28] Patients with advanced NSCLC treated with best supportive care alone had a median survival of 4–5 months.[57] Chemotherapy for advanced NSCLC was also shown to improve quality of life and be cost-effective.[58,59] Systemic chemotherapy for advanced disease is now the standard of care for patients of good performance status.[60] Diffusing the negative impression of chemotherapy from the community has been difficult, and recent studies have shown reluctance on the part of primary care providers to encourage treatment for metastatic lung cancer as compared with other solid tumours. Epidemiological data have also shown that racial identity and socioeconomic status can affect whether patients are offered chemotherapy for their lung cancer.[61,62] Specific groups such as poor performance status patients, and need for palliative radiation, will be covered in a later section.

TREATMENT REGIMENS

Platinum-containing doublets

Single-agent activity against lung cancer has been demonstrated for many agents but early studies demonstrated the role of cisplatin and carboplatin in the treatment of NSCLC when combined with other active agents. Some of these studies are summarized in Table 4.2. These studies showed that there was no statistically significant difference between any of the platinum-containing doublets in activity or survival.[63–66] The consensus of opinion supports the use of the platinum-containing doublet as the first-line treatment in advanced NSCLC.[60,67] Side effect profile and

Table 4.2 Selected cooperative group trials of chemoradiation therapy with unresectable stage III NSCLC

Trial	Median survival (months)	3–year survival (%)
CALGB 8433 (radiotherapy)	9.6	10
CALGB (sequential chemoradiotherapy)	13.7	24
RTOG 9104 (concurrent chemoradiotherapy)	14.6	31
RTOG 9410 (sequential chemoradiotherapy)	14.6	31
RTOG 9410 (concurrent chemoradiotherapy)	17.0	37
SWOG 9504	26.0	37

Reproduced with permission from Curran WJ Jr: Treatment of locally advanced non-small cell lung cancer: what we have and have not learned over the past decade. Semin Oncol 2005; 32(Suppl 3): S2–S5. © Elsevier.

regional differences often account for the preference of one regimen or another. Commonly used regimens in Europe include cisplatin 100 mg/m^2 IV day 1/gemcitabine 1250 mg/m^2 IV day 1 and 8 every 21 days. In France, cisplatin 120 mg/m^2 day 1/vinorelbine 30 mg/m^2 IV on day 1 and 8 every 28 days is often used, while in the US carboplatin AUC 6 day 1/paclitaxel (175 mg/m^2) given day 1 every 21 days. Other common regimens include carboplatin AUC 5 IV day 1/gemcitabine 1000 mg/m^2 IV days 1 and 8 every 21 days, cisplatin 75 mg/m^2 IV day 1/docetaxel 75 mg/m^2 IV day 1 every 21 days, carboplatin AUC 6 IV day 1/docetaxel 75 mg/m^2 IV day 1.[60]

Carboplatin vs. cisplatin

The question of which platinum agent is more effective has also been examined. Studies have shown a slight survival advantage for cisplatin, but at the expense of greater toxicity.[65,68] The current consensus is that while cisplatin might have slightly more activity in NSCLC, any difference between cisplatin and carboplatin is small, and treatment choices should be made on an individual case basis and guided by side effect profile.[63,68] For patients who cannot tolerate a platinum doublet, non-platinum doublets have been shown to have activity, most notably paclitaxel/gemcitabine, and gemcitabine 1200 mg/m^2 IV day 1 and 8/vinorelbine 30 mg/m^2 IV day 1 and 8 every 21 days. These agents could be considered if patients are unable to tolerate platinum but are otherwise fit for chemotherapy.[60] Studies examining the role of triplet chemotherapy have not shown increased response rates, but have shown increased toxicity from treatment.[69] Table 4.3 lists the doublet regimens studied in randomized trials showing similar results. [63–66] There is no evidence at this time to support triplet therapy with standard chemotherapy agents outside a clinic trial. Improvements on the platinum-containing doublet invariably turned to targeted agents and away from traditional cytotoxic chemotherapeutic agents.

Advances in first-line therapy

The addition of bevacizumab, a monoclonal antibody to vascular endothelial growth factor, to carboplatin and paclitaxel resulted in a significantly improved survival and response compared with chemotherapy alone.[70] The response rate was increased from 15% to 35%, and the median survival increased from 10.3 to 12.3 months. The treatment was well tolerated, but certain subgroups, including patients with squamous cell cancer and large central tumours, were more likely to suffer from severe airway haemorrhage.[70] Confirmatory studies with other

Table 4.3 Phase III trials of chemotherapy regimens for non-small cell lung cancer

Trial	Regimen	Patients	Response rate (%)	Median survival (months)	1-year survival (%)
ECOG[63]	Paclitaxel/cisplatin	305	21	7.8	31
	Gemcitabine/cisplatin	288	22	8.1	36
	Docetaxel/cisplatin	289	17	7.4	31
	Paclitaxel/carboplatin	290	17	8.1	34
ILCSG[64]	Vinorelbine/cisplatin	201	30	9.5	37
	Gemcitabine/cisplatin	205	30	9.8	37
	Paclitaxel/carboplatin	201	32	9.9	43
Tax-326[65]	Cisplatin/vinorelbine	404	25	10.1	41
	Cisplatin/docetaxel	408	32	11.3	46
	Carboplatin/docetaxel	406	24	9.4	38
SWOG[66]	Paclitaxel/carboplatin	206	25	8	38
	Vinorelbine/cisplatin	202	28	8	36

ECOG, Eastern Cooperative Oncology Group; ILCSG, Italian Lung Cancer Study Group; SWOG, Southwest Oncology Group.

chemotherapy regimens are ongoing. Bevacizumab has recently been licensed in the US for use with carboplatin and taxol as first-line therapy, and an application has been submitted in Europe. Currently, this treatment option should be considered for patients of good performance status who have a non-squamous lung cancer without a history of brain metastasis or bulky central tumour. A treatment algorithm for first-line treatment with systemic chemotherapy is shown in Figure 4.5.[60] A number of other novel targeted agents are currently under evaluation in the first-line setting including other antibodies and small molecule inhibitors of angiogenesis, EGFR and other signalling pathways.

Second-line therapy

The effectiveness of first-line therapy in lung cancer naturally led many to investigate the effectiveness of these agents after first-line treatment. The first agent to be approved for second-line therapy in NSCLC was docetaxel. When docetaxel 75 mg/m^2 IV every 21 days was compared with best supportive care it was found to improve survival rates and quality of life.[71] Another study demonstrated increased effectiveness vs. other known agents in the second-line setting.[72] These studies established docetaxel as the standard of care in patients who had previously

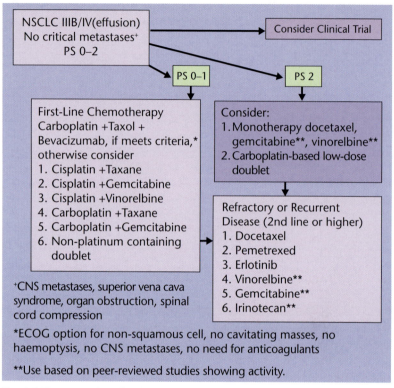

Fig. 4.5 Treatment algorithm for stage IIIB/IV non-small cell lung cancer (NSCLC) (Modified algorithm based on data from ref. 60).

received chemotherapy and as the control arm for future studies in second-line patients. Recently, the multi-targeted antifolate drug, pemetrexed, which had shown activity in mesothelioma, was also shown to have activity in NSCLC, with a response rate of 15.8%.[73,74] Vitamin B12 and folate supplementation has been shown to decrease toxicity, and is now standard.[75] When compared directly with docetaxel, the response rates and survival were identical, but the toxicity profile favoured pemetrexed. Pemetrexed has emerged as a legitimate alternative to docetaxel as a second-line agent.[76]

Gemcitabine 1000 mg/m^2 IV on days 1, 8 and 15 every 28 days and vinorelbine 25 mg/m^2 IV days 1 and 8 every 21 days have both been shown to have activity in the first-line treatment of NSCLC, but they are not as well studied as docetaxel and pemetrexed in the second-line setting. Given their known toxicity profiles, they may be considered for treatment if docetaxel and premetrexed are not an option, although they are not licensed for this indication.[60]

EGFR antagonists

The EGFR antagonists have become an important tool in the treatment of lung cancer. These small molecules have changed the way that subtypes of lung cancer are treated, as well as providing another option for second- and third-line treatment for patients with NSCLC.[77] Gefitinib was the first EGFR inhibitor to show promise in clinical trials; however, its initial phase II responses did not appear to result in survival benefit in large phase III trials.[78] The addition of gefitinib to standard chemotherapy did not result in a survival advantage.[79,80] In retrospect, this was not surprising as there is no compelling evidence that three drugs are better than two in the treatment of NSCLC. Similar studies with erlotinib also failed to show a benefit.[81,82] Phase II studies of gefitinib as second- or third-line therapy (IDEAL 1 & 2) yielded similar response rates to those seen for conventional second-line therapy.[71,83,84] Phase III studies of gefitinib and erlotinib as second-line therapy have shown different outcomes. The ISEL trial randomized 1,692 previously treated patients to gefitinib or placebo. Response rates showed a significantly higher response rate for gefitinib, but no difference in survival.[85] A similarly designed study by the National Cancer Institute of Canada (NCIC) comparing erlotinib with placebo in 731 patients reported a significant survival advantage for erlotinib.[84]

The similarities between the treatments and trials have been widely discussed.[86] Erlotinib is now licensed for the second-line and third-line treatment of NSCLC in the US and in Europe.

Known side effects include diarrhoea and rash, as well as a rare incidence of interstitial lung disease, but overall the EGFR inhibitors are better tolerated than cytotoxic chemotherapy.[77] Subgroup analysis revealed that certain groups – patients with adenocarcinoma, women, non-smokers and patients of East Asian decent – were more likely to respond to the EGFR inhibitors.[87] These findings and the anecdotal findings of clinicians that some patients had a dramatic response to the EGFR inhibitors led to the discovery that patients with EGFR mutations in the ATP binding pocket of the intracellular domain of EGFR had a better response to gefitinib, and later erlotinib.[87–89] Currently, clinical trials are investigating the role of EGFR inhibitors in first-line treatment for clinical subgroups as well as patients who harbour the EGFR receptor mutation, and in maintenance therapy for patients responding to first-line chemotherapy.

EGFR copy number and protein expression seem to be important determinants of survival benefit with EGFR inhibitors, the importance of receptor mutation status is less clear.[90]

ELDERLY PATIENTS

Lung cancer is more common in elderly patients. The most recent data from the Surveillance, Epidemiology and End Results programme show that 67% of patients were over 65 years of age at diagnosis (available at http://seer.cancer.gov). The decision on whether to offer treatment to elderly patients, commonly accepted as >65–70 years, will be influenced by a number of factors including performance status and comorbidity. There is a concern that age-related decrease in organ function will increase the risk of significant toxicity in older patients. In addition, older patients have a higher incidence of comorbidity. While a number of comorbidity scores have been devised, these correlate poorly with performance status, the current standard tool used to assess suitability for chemotherapy, and how to incorporate these scores into decision making processes is unclear.

Approximately 80% of lung cancer patients over 65 years are not offered chemotherapy,[61] yet subgroup analysis from CALG B[91] and the NSCLC meta-analysis[28] revealed no impact of age on survival. However, patients included in clinical trials are often highly selected and may not be representative of the general population.

A number of studies have looked specifically at the effect of age on outcome. The use of platinum-containing doublets in this group is controversial. Although some studies indicate that the platinum doublets have a similar activity in this group,[92] they have also found higher toxicity in elderly patients on these regimens.

Monotherapy with non-platinum agents such as vinorelbine was found to have moderate activity in patients aged 70 years and older in the Elderly Lung Cancer Vinorelbine Group Study (ELVIS). In this study 161 patients ≥70 years of age were randomized to single-agent vinorelbine or best supportive care. One-year survival (32% vs. 14%) and quality of life were significantly better for the chemotherapy-treated patients.[93]

The role of combination therapy has also been examined. The Multicentre Italian Lung Cancer in the Elderly Study (MILES) randomized nearly 700 patients to either vinorelbine, gemcitabine or vinorelbine + gemcitabine.[94] There was no advantage to combination therapy over single-agent treatment and toxicity was higher. Activity has been seen with other agents, such as gemcitabine, docetaxel and paclitaxel.[60]

Subset analysis of a number of phase III studies has shown no difference in outcome for elderly patients.[63,65] The recent guidelines from the American Society for Clinical Oncology for the treatment of elderly patients with advanced NSCLC recommend single-agent chemotherapy, although these decisions should be individualized.[5] Studies with fractionated chemotherapy doses have shown promising results. The demonstrable activity and manageable toxicity of targeted therapies make them prime targets for evaluation in elderly patients.

POOR PERFORMANCE STATUS PATIENTS

Patients with a poor performance status represent a significant part of oncology practice. Many studies tend to include these with elderly patients, although clearly they are a distinct group. Several recent trials comparing combination regimens have reported subset analysis of patients with poor performance status. The Eastern Cooperative Oncology Group (ECOG) 1594 study comparing four platinum-based doublets stopped accrual of performance status 2 patients early in the trial due to the high rate of toxicity and early deaths. However, subsequent analysis of the patients treated showed that the majority of deaths were due to disease and not treatment related.[95] Similarly, a study from the Spanish Lung Cancer Group comparing cisplatin-based doublet and triplet regimens with non-platinum sequential doublet regimens reported a much worse outcome for patients with performance status 2.[69] Similar findings have been reported in subset analysis from large studies carried out by the EORTC and by the Hellenic Cooperative Oncology Group.[96,97] The current American Society of Clinical Oncology guidelines recommend single-agent chemotherapy for patients with performance status 2.[5]

SMALL CELL CARCINOMA OF THE LUNG

Our understanding of the optimum management of small cell lung cancer has improved significantly over the last 10 years. Unlike NSCLC, the role for surgery has been limited given the rapid doubling time of the cancer.[98,99] Surgery for small cell lung cancer had been avoided for years, until recent data described some success in resecting stage IB localized tumours followed by adjuvant treatment with chemotherapy.[98] Generally resections of patients with small cell lung cancer are discovered retrospectively when resecting what appears to be NSCLC clinically.[100] The opportunities for treatment in this manner are limited, and the majority of small cell lung cancer is treated with a combination of chemotherapy and radiation.

Limited stage small cell lung cancer

Treatment of limited stage small cell lung cancer with combination chemotherapy has been the standard of care since the superiority of the etoposide/cisplatin regimen was demonstrated.[101,102]

The gold standard chemotherapy for patients with good prognosis disease is a platinum-based regimen, typically cisplatin/etoposide (PE). Many studies report a median survival of 17–18 months with cisplatin combined with radiotherapy, significantly higher than most reported for anthracycline-based therapy.[103] A recent comparison of PE with cyclophosphamide/epirubicin/vincristine (CEV)[102] showed that overall survival was significantly better for those patients randomized to receive PE (10.2 vs. 7.8 months, p=0.0004), and a recent overview of US National Cancer Institute-sponsored trials in extensive stage small cell cancer demonstrated that platinum-containing regimens do impart a relatively modest survival advantage when compared with non-platinum regimens.[104] It was also noted that the baseline survival had improved, probably due to improvements in supportive care. A further meta-analysis of 19 trials published between 1981 and 1999 showed a significant survival advantage for patients receiving platinum-based chemotherapy when compared with those not receiving this drug.[105]

Given the chemosensitivity of small cell lung cancer, and the high response rates, many studies have used growth factor support to intensify the treatment administered. The results of many of these studies have been conflicting. There is no clear role for dose intensification in small cell lung cancer, although maintaining the dose intensity of standard treatment is very important.[106–110]

Extensive stage small cell lung cancer

Small cell lung cancer outside of the thorax is treated with chemotherapy alone and platinum-based chemotherapy is the treatment of choice.[104] Studies have noted that substitution of carboplatin is a reasonable alterative if toxicity is a major concern.[111] Response rates to chemotherapy are 60–80% in extensive stage, and median life expectancy is 8–13 months.[100] A recent study comparing the newer combination of cisplatin/irinotecan with PE showed a significant survival benefit in a Japanese population of patients (median survival 12.8 vs. 9.4 months);[112] however a larger confirmatory study failed to show a difference in outcome.[113]

Many patients with small cell lung cancer also have a poor perform-ance status and/or a number of adverse prognostic factors. Outcomes for these patients are poor. Treatment approaches have included the use of low-dose high-frequency regimens,[107] abbreviated chemotherapy fol-lowed by radiotherapy[108] or reduced-dose combination therapies.[109] A study comparing 3-weekly chemotherapy with treatment given as required for symptom control showed an improvement in quality of life in those receiving regular treatment.[110] Other studies have tested inten-sive one-drug or two-drug regimens. A UK Medical Research Council study demonstrated similar efficacy of an etoposide and vincristine reg-imen and a four-drug regimen.[114] The latter had a greater risk of toxici-ty and early death but was superior in palliation of symptoms and psy-chological distress. Studies comparing an oral treatment with single-agent oral etoposide with combination therapy[115,116] showed that the overall response rate and survival were significantly worse in the oral etoposide arm with a suggestion of an increased number of early deaths in patients receiving this treatment. More recently, a randomized com-parison of single-agent carboplatin (AUC 6) with cyclophosphamide, doxorubicin and vincristine (CAV) in patients with Karnofsky perform-ance ≤50 and a prognostic score indicator of a 1-year survival ≤15% showed that median and overall survivals were similar for both arms, with less toxicity in the carboplatin arm.[117] At present, a standard ther-apy for patients with poor prognosis small cell lung cancer is a combina-tion of carboplatin plus etoposide, and single-agent carboplatin for those with very poor prognosis (e.g. ≤20% survival at 1 year).

Treatment of relapsed or refractory disease

Patients who do not respond or who relapse within 3 months are consid-ered refractory to treatment. For sensitive patients (those patients with a durable response beyond 3 months), the same induction regimen can be used for retreatment. A recent phase III trial demonstrated that the addi-tion of oral topotecan to best supportive care significantly increases over-all survival (median overall survival 25.9 weeks vs. 13.9 weeks for best supportive care, p=0.01) and better symptom control compared with best supportive care alone in patients with relapsed small cell lung cancer. This is the first randomized trial comparing chemotherapy with best supportive care in relapsed small cell lung cancer.[118] A randomized comparison of topotecan vs. CAV in 211 patients with small cell lung cancer who had relapsed at least 60 days after completion of first-line therapy showed no difference in response rate or survival between treatment arms, but patients receiving topotecan had better symptom control. Toxicity in both arms was considerable.[119] An early randomized phase II trial and preliminary results from a phase III study confirm that oral topotecan has activity and tolerability similar to IV topotecan in chemosensitive small cell lung cancer and offers patients a convenient alternative to intravenous therapy.[120,121] Intravenous topotecan is the first agent to be approved in Europe and in the US that is specifically indicated for the treatment of relapsed small cell lung cancer for which re-treatment with the first-line regimen is not considered appropriate. A licence application for the oral formulation of topotecan is planned.

A number of other new drugs are being evaluated and showing promise in early studies; these are reviewed in detail elsewhere.[122]

Radiotherapy for limited stage small cell lung cancer

Radiotherapy plays an important role in the management of limited stage small cell lung cancer. Randomized trials have shown that thoracic radiotherapy and prophylactic cranial irradiation improve both tumour control and overall survival. Combination chemotherapy alone is associated with intrathoracic failure rates of 75–90%. The addition of thoracic irradiation reduces the risk of intrathoracic failure to 30–60%.[123–125]

Two meta-analyses showed a statistically significant advantage associated with the addition of thoracic radiotherapy to chemotherapy.[126,127] Essential questions related to the optimization of thoracic radiotherapy remain unanswered. In particular, the optimal radiotherapy dose, fractionation and treatment volume have not been well defined.

Historically, small cell lung cancer was treated with lower doses of radiation than NSCLC because patients receive initial chemotherapy, and small cell lung cancer is considered to be a radiosensitive disease. However, while improved chemotherapy increases the control of distant metastases, low-dose schedules such as 30 Gy in 10 fractions are associated with a high frequency of local failure. Retrospective studies suggest that thoracic radiotherapy doses of 50 Gy or more can translate into improved progression-free survival but an impact on overall survival has yet to be demonstrated. Doses similar to the doses given for non-small cell cancers may be necessary to improve both local control and overall survival.

Conventional radiotherapy fractionation can be modified by hyperfractionation (radiotherapy given more than once a day) and/or acceleration (shortening of the overall treatment time). Studies on small cell lung cancer cell lines showed a small shoulder on radiation survival curves and low surviving fractions at 2 Gy. These observations suggest that small cell lung cancer may be sensitive to, and thus benefit from, the lower doses used in hyperfractionated radiotherapy. Five-year survival rates greater than 20% are reported with twice-daily radiotherapy with concurrent chemotherapy.[128–130] A landmark study by Turrisi et al compared 45 Gy given either twice daily (1.5 Gy per fraction) over 3 weeks or once daily (1.8 Gy per fraction) over 5 weeks.[128] Radiation was given concurrently starting with the first cycle of chemotherapy. Twice daily radiotherapy improved overall 5-year survival (26% vs. 16% in the once-daily arm) but increased the rate of grade 3/4 radiation oesophagitis (32% vs. 16% in the once-daily arm).

Chemotherapy and radiotherapy can be delivered concurrently, sequentially or as alternating treatments. When comparing the results of randomized controlled trials, it appears that the best results have been seen with early concurrent thoracic radiotherapy.[129–131] The 20% 5-year survival milestone has generally been achieved with early thoracic irradiation. A Japanese study comparing sequential to concurrent chemoradiotherapy has demonstrated the superiority of concurrent chemoradiotherapy.[129] In 2004 two meta-analyses evaluated the timing of thoracic radiation in combined modality therapy. In the Cochrane review[132] there was no significant 2- or 3-year overall survival benefit in favour of early (defined as starting within 30 days of initiation of chemotherapy) vs. late thoracic radiotherapy with either cisplatin-based (odds ratio 0.73, 95% confidence interval 0.5–1.03, p=0.07) or non-cisplatin-based chemotherapy (odds ratio 1.97, 95% confidence interval 1.10–3.53, p=0.42). There was a 5-year survival benefit in favour of early thoracic radiotherapy and cisplatin-based chemotherapy (odds ratio 0.64, 95% confidence interval 0.44–0.92, p=0.02). In contrast in the Fried et al. meta-analysis[133] studies using platinum-based chemotherapy had a 2-year overall survival benefit for early (defined as prior to 9 weeks after initiation of chemotherapy) compared with late thoracic radiotherapy of 9.8% (95% confidence interval 3.8%–15.9%, p=0.002), favouring early thoracic radiotherapy. The new concept of SER (Start of any treatment to End of Radiotherapy) also supports early thoracic radiotherapy.[134] The study suggested that with cisplatin-based regimens the ideal SER was ≤40 days, supporting the use of a radiotherapy regimen given concurrently with the first cycle of chemotherapy or starting with the second cycle of chemotherapy providing the overall treatment time is short (e.g. 30 fractions twice daily or 15 fractions once daily).

Prophylactic cranial irradiation (PCI) also plays an important role in the management of this disease. Patients whose cancer can be controlled have a 60% actuarial risk of developing brain metastasis within 2–3 years after starting treatment. This risk can be decreased by 50% by the administration of PCI. A meta-analysis of seven randomized controlled trials evaluating the role of PCI in patients in complete remission after chemotherapy reported improvement in brain recurrence, disease-free survival and overall survival with the addition of PCI.[135] Prospective studies have shown that patients treated with PCI do not have significantly worse neuropsychological function than patients not treated.[135,136] The EULINT PCI trial randomized 700 patients to high-dose (36 Gy in 18 fractions) or standard-dose (25 Gy in 10 fractions) radiotherapy to the whole brain. The first results are awaited in 2007. The role of PCI in extensive stage disease has been the result of a recent randomized trial, the results of which will be available in 2007.

REFERENCES

1. Early lung cancer detection: summary and conclusions. Am Rev Respir Dis 1984; 130(4) : 565–570.
2. Jett JR, Midthun DE: Screening for lung cancer: current status and future directions: Thomas A. Neff lecture. Chest 2004; 125(5 Suppl): 158S–162S.
3. Mountain CF: Revisions in the International System for Staging Lung Cancer. Chest 1997; 111(6): 1710–1717.
4. Sihoe AD, Yim AP: Lung cancer staging. J Surg Res 2004; 117: 92–106.
5. Pfister DG, Johnson DH et al: American Society of Clinical Oncology treatment of unresectable non-small-cell lung cancer guideline: update 2003. J Clin Oncol 2004; 22: 330–353.
6. Mentzer SJ: Mediastinoscopy, thoracoscopy, and video-assisted thoracic surgery in the diagnosis and staging of lung cancer. Hematol Oncol Clin North Am 1997; 11(3): 435–447.
7. Pass HI: Mediastinal staging 2005: pictures, scopes, and scalpels. Semin Oncol 2005; 32(3): 269–278.
8. Mentzer SJ: Thoracoscopy and video assisted thoracic surgery. Current Medicine Philadelphia, DC, 1994.
9. Surmont V, van Klaveren RJ, Goor C: Lessons to learn from EORTC study 08981: A feasibility study of induction chemoradiotherapy followed by surgical resection for stage IIIB NSCLC. Lung Cancer 2006 Oct 25; [Epub ahead of print].
10. Toloza EM, Harpole L, Detterbeck F, McCrory DC: Invasive staging of non-small cell lung cancer: A review of the current evidence. Chest 2003; 123(1 Suppl): 157S–166S.
11. Detterbeck FC, Falen S, et al: Seeking a home for a PET, part 1: Defining the appropriate place for positron emission tomography imaging in the diagnosis of pulmonary nodules or masses. Chest 2004; 125(6): 2294–2299.
12. Detterbeck FC, Falen S, et al: Seeking a home for a PET, part 2: Defining the appropriate place for positron emission tomography imaging in the staging of patients with suspected lung cancer. Chest 2004; 125(6): 2300–2308.
13. Herder GJ, Breuer RH, et al: Positron emission tomography scans can detect radiographically occult lung cancer in the central airways. J Clin Oncol 2001; 19(22): 4271–4272.

14. Lardinois D, Weder W, et al: Staging of non-small-cell lung cancer with integrated positron-emission tomography and computed tomography. N Engl J Med 2003; 348(25): 2500–2508.
15. Toloza EM, Harpole L, McCrory DC: Noninvasive staging of non-small cell lung cancer: a review of the current evidence. Chest 2003; 123(1 Suppl): 137S–146S.
16. Detterbeck FC, Vansteenkiste JF, et al: Seeking a home for a PET, part 3: Emerging applications of positron emission tomography imaging in the management of patients with lung cancer. Chest 2004; 126(5): 1656–1666.
17. Herder GJ, Kramer H, et al: Traditional versus up-front [18F] fluorodeoxyglucose-positron emission tomography staging of non-small-cell lung cancer: a Dutch cooperative randomized study. J Clin Oncol 2006; 24(12): 1800–1806.
18. Marom EM, Erasmus JJ, Patz EF: Lung cancer and positron emission tomography with fluorodeoxyglucose. Lung Cancer 2000; 28(3): 187–202.
19. Dunagan D, Chin R Jr, et al: Staging by positron emission tomography predicts survival in patients with non-small cell lung cancer. Chest 2001; 119(2): 333–339.
20. Zelen M: Keynote address on biostatistics and data retrieval. Cancer Chemother Rep 1973; 4(2): 31–42.
21. Mountain CF. A new international staging system for lung cancer. Chest 1986; 89: 225–233.
22. Cerny T, Blair V, Anderson H, et al: Pretreatment prognostic factors and scoring system in 407 small-cell lung cancer patients. Int J Cancer 1987; 39: 146–149.
23. Rawson MS, Peto J: An overview of prognostic factors in small cell lung cancer, a report from the subcommittee for the management of lung cancer of the UKCCCR. Br J Cancer 1990; 61: 597–604.
24. Paesmans M, Sculier JP, et al: Prognostic factors for patients with small cell lung cancer: analysis of a series of 763 patients included in 4 consecutive prospective clinical trials with a minimum follow-up of 5 years. Cancer 2000: 89(3): 523–533.
25. Albain KS, Crowley JJ, Livingston RB: Long-term survival and toxicity in small cell lung cancer. Expanded Southwest Oncology Group experience. Chest 1991; 99(6): 1425–1432.
26. Farray DF, Mirkovic N, Albain KS: Multimodality therapy for stage III non-small cell lung cancer. J Clin Oncol 2005; 23(14): 3257–3269.
27. PORT Meta-analysis Trialists Group: Postoperative radiotherapy in non-small cell lung cancer: Review and meta-analysis of individual patient data from nine randomized controlled trials. Lancet 1998; 352(9124):257–263.
28. NSCLC Collaborative Group: Chemotherapy in non-small cell lung cancer: a meta-analysis using updated data on individual patients from 52 randomized clinical trials. Non-small Cell Lung Cancer Collaborative Group. BMJ 1995; 311(7010): 899–909.
29. Arriagada R, Bergman B, et al: Cisplatin-based adjuvant chemotherapy in patients with completely resected non-small-call lung cancer. N Engl J Med 2004; 350: 351–360.
30. Winton TL, Livingston R et al: Prospective randomized trial of adjuvant vinorelbine and cisplatin in completely resected stage IB and stage II non small cell lung cancer. Intergroup JBR10. J Clin Oncol 2004; 22(14S):7018.

31. Douillard JY, Rosell R, et al: ANITA: Phase II adjuvant vinorelbine (N) and cisplatin (P) versus observation in completely resected non small cell lung cancer. J Clin Oncol 2005; 23(16S): 7013.
32. Hotta K, Matsuo K, et al: Role of adjuvant chemotherapy in patients with resected non-small cell lung cancer: reappraisal with a meta-analysis of randomized controlled trials. J Clin Oncol 2004; 22: 3860–3867.
33. Sedrakyan A, van Der Meulen J, et al: Postoperative chemotherapy for non-small cell lung cancer: a systematic review and meta-analysis. J Thorac Cardiovasc Surg 2004; 128: 414–419.
34. Juergens RA, Brahmer JR: Adjuvant treatment in non-small cell lung cancer: where are we now? J Natl Compr Cancer Netw 2006; 4: 595–600.
35. Domont J, Soria JC, Le Chevalier T: Adjuvant chemotherapy in early-stage non-small cell lung cancer. Semin Oncol 2005; 32(3): 279–283.
36. Strauss GM, Herndon JE, Maddaus MA, et al: Adjuvant chemotherapy in stage IB non-small cell lung cancer: Update of Cancer and Leukemia Group B (CALGB) protocol 9633. J Clin Oncol 2006; 24(18S): 7007.
37. Wada H, Miyahara R, et al: Postoperative adjuvant chemotherapy with PVM (cisplatin+vindesine+mitomycin C) and UFT (uracil+tegagul) in resected stage I-II SNCLC (non-small cell lung cancer): a randomized clinical trial. Eur J Cardiothorac Surg 1999; 15: 438–443.
38. Endo C, Saito Y, et al: A randomized trial of postoperative UFT therapy in p stage I, II non-small cell lung cancer: North-east Japan Study Group for Lung cancer Surgery. J Lung Cancer 2003; 40: 181–186.
39. Kato H, Ichinose Y, et al: A randomized trial of adjuvant chemotherapy with uracil-tegafur for adenocarcinoma of the lung. N Engl J Med 2004; 350: 1713–1721.
40. Roth J, Fossella F, et al: A randomized trial comparing preoperative chemotherapy and surgery with surgery alone in respectable Stage IIIa NSCLC. J Natl Cancer Inst 1994; 86; 973–980.
41. Rossell R, Gomez-Codina J, et al: A randomized trial comparing preoperative chemotherapy + surgery with surgery alone in patients with NSCLC. New Engl J Med 1994; 330: 153–158.
42. Pass H, Pogrehniak H, et al: Randomised trial of neoadjuvant therapy for lung cancer; interim analysis. Ann Thoracic Surgery 1992; 53: 992–998.
43. Depierre A, Milleron B, et al: Peroperative chemotherapy followed by surgery compared to primary surgery in respectable NSCLC. J Clin Oncology 2002; 20: 247–253.
44. Dillman RO, Herndon J, et al: Improved survival in stage III non-small-cell lung cancer: Seven-year follow-up of Cancer and Leukemia Group B (CALGB) 8433 trial. J Natl Cancer Inst 1996; 88: 1210–1215.
45. Sause W, Kolear P, et al: Final results of phase III trial in regionally advanced unresectable non-small cell lung cancer: Radiation Therapy Oncology Group, Eastern Cooperative Oncology Group, Southwest Oncology Group. Chest 2000; 117: 358–364.
46. Le Chevalier T, Arraigade R, et al: Radiotherapy alone versus combined chemotherapy and radiotherapy in unresectable non-small cell lung carcinoma. Lung Cancer 1994; 10(Suppl 1): S239–S244.
47. Furuse K, Fukuoka M, et al: Phase III study of concurrent versus sequential thoracic radiotherapy in combination with mitomycin, vindesine, and cisplatin in unresectable stage III non-small-cell lung cancer. J Clin Oncol 1999; 17: 2692–2699.

48. Pierre F, Perol M, et al: A randomized phase III trial of sequential chemotherapy versus concurrent chemo-radiotherapy in locally advanced non-small cell lung cancer (GLOT-GFPC NPC 96-01 study). Proc Am Soc Clin Oncol 2001; 20: 312a (abstr 1246).

49. Curran WJ, Scott CB, et al: Long-term benefit is observed in a phase III comparison of sequential versus concurrent chemo-radiation for patients with unresected stage III NSCLC: TROG 9410. Proc Am Soc Clin Oncol 2003; 22: 621 (abstr 2499).

50. Zatloukal P, Petruzelka L, et al: Concurrent versus sequential chemoradio-therapy with cisplatin and vinorelbine in locally advanced non-small cell lung cancer: A randomized study. Lung Cancer 2004; 46: 87–98.

51. Schaake-Koning C, van der Bogaert W, et al: Effects of concomitant cisplatin and radiotherapy on inoperable non-small cell lung cancer. N Engl J Med 1992; 326: 524–530.

52. Gandara DR, Chansky K, et al: Consolidation docetaxel after concurrent chemoradiotherapy in stage IIIB non-small-cell lung cancer: phase II Southwest Oncology Group Study S9504. J Clin Oncol 2003; 21(10): 2004–2010.

53. Albain K, Swann R, Rusch V: Phase III trial of concurrent chemotherapy and radiotherapy (CT/RT) vs CT/RT followed by surgical resection for stage IIIA (pN2) NSCLC: outcomes update of RTOG 9309. Proc Am Soc Clin Oncol 2005; 23: 16S: # 7014.

54. Ruebe C, Riesenbeck D, et al: Neoadjuvant chemotherapy followed by pre-operative radiochemotherapy (hfRTCT) plus surgery or surgery plus postop-erative radiotherapy in stage III non-small cell lung cancer: Results of a ran-domized phase III trial of the German Lung Cancer Cooperative Group. Int J Radiat Oncol Biol Phys 2004; 60(1 suppl): S130.

55. Van Meerbeeck JP, Kramer G, Van Schil PE et al: A randomized trial of radi-cal surgery versus thoracic radiotherapy in patients with stage IIIA–N2 non-small cell lung cancer after response to induction chemotherapy (EORTC 08941). J Clin Oncol 2005; 23(16S): 7015.

56. Rusch VW, Giroux DJ, et al: Induction chemoradiation and surgical resec-tion for non-small cell lung carcinomas of the superior sulcus; Initial results of South West Oncology Group trial 9416 (intergroup trial 0160). J Thorac Cardiovasc Surg 2001; 121: 472–483.

57. Johnson DH: Chemotherapy for metastatic non-small-cell lung cancer—can that dog hunt? J Natl Cancer Inst 1993; 85(10): 766–767.

58. Evans WK, Will BP, et al: The economics of lung cancer management in Canada. Lung Cancer 1996; 14(1): 19–29.

59. Cullen MH, Billingham LJ, et al: Mitomycin, ifosfamide, and cisplatin in unresectable non-small-cell lung cancer: effects on survival and quality of life. J Clin Oncol 1999; 17(10): 3188–3194.

60. Milton DT, Miller VA: Advances in cytotoxic chemotherapy for the treat-ment of metastatic or recurrent non-small cell lung cancer. Semin Oncol 2005; 32(3): 299–314.

61. Earle CC, Venditti LN, et al: Who gets chemotherapy for metastatic lung cancer? Chest 2000; 117(5): 1239–1246.

62. Earle CC, Neumann PJ, et al: Impact of referral patterns on the use of chemotherapy for lung cancer. J Clin Oncol 2002; 20(7): 1786–1792.

63. Schiller JH, Harrington D, et al: Comparison of four chemotherapy regi-mens for advanced non-small-cell lung cancer. N Engl J Med 2002; 346(2): 92–98.

64. Scagliotti GV, Fossati R, et al: Randomized study of adjuvant chemotherapy for completely resected stage I, II, or IIIA non-small-cell lung cancer. J Natl Cancer Inst 2003; 95(19):1453–1461.
65. Fossella F, Pereira JR, et al: Randomized, multinational, phase III study of docetaxel plus platinum combinations versus vinorelbine plus cisplatin for advanced non-small-cell lung cancer: The TAX 326 study group. J Clin Oncol 2003; 21(16): 3016–3024.
66. Kelly K, Crowley J, et al: Randomized phase III trial of paclitaxel plus carboplatin versus vinorelbine plus cisplatin in the treatment of patients with advanced non-small-cell lung cancer: A Southwest Oncology Group trial. J Clin Oncol 2001; 19(13): 3210–3218.
67. Laskin JJ, Sandler AB: First-line treatment for advanced non-small-cell lung cancer. Oncology (Williston Park) 2005; 19(13): 1671–1676; discussion 1678–1680.
68. Rosell R, Gatzemeier U, et al: Phase III randomized trial comparing paclitaxel/carboplatin with paclitaxel/cisplatin in patients with advanced non-small-cell lung cancer: a cooperative multinational trial. Ann Oncol 2002; 13(10): 1539–1549.
69. Alberola V, Camps C, et al: Cisplatin plus gemcitabine versus a cisplatin-based triplet versus nonplatinum sequential doublets in advanced non-small-cell lung cancer: A Spanish Lung Cancer Group phase III randomized trial. J Clin Oncol 2003; 21: 3207–3213.
70. Sandler AB, Gray R, et al: Randomized phase II/III trial of paclitaxel plus carboplatin with our without bevacizumab in patients with advanced non-squamous non-small cell lung cancer: An Eastern Cooperative Oncology Group (ECOG) Trial—E4599. J Clin Oncol 2005; 23(16S): 4.
71. Shepherd FA, Dancey J, Ramlau R, et al: Prospective randomized trial of docetaxel versus best supportive care in patients with non-small-cell lung cancer previously treated with platinum-based chemotherapy. J Clin Oncol 2000; 18(10): 2095–2103.
72. Fossella FV, DeVore R, et al: Randomized phase III trial of docetaxel versus vinorelbine or ifosfamide in patients with advanced non-small-cell lung cancer previously treated with platinum-containing chemotherapy regimens. The TAX 320 Non-Small Cell Lung Cancer Study Group. J Clin Oncol 2000; 18(12): 2354–2362.
73. Clarke SJ, Abratt R, et al: Phase II trial of pemetrexed disodium (ALIMTA, LY231514) in chemotherapy-naive patients with advanced non-small-cell lung cancer. Ann Oncol 2002; 13(5): 737–741.
74. Smit EF, Mattson K, et al: ALIMTA (pemetrexed disodium) as second-line treatment of non-small-cell lung cancer: A phase II study. Ann Oncol 2003; 14(3): 455–460.
75. Bajetta E, Celio L, et al: Phase II study of pemetrexed disodium (Alimta) administered with oral folic acid in patients with advanced gastric cancer. Ann Oncol 2003; 14(10): 1543–1548.
76. Hanna N, Shepherd FA, et al: Randomized phase III trial of pemetrexed versus docetaxel in patients with non-small-cell lung cancer previously treated with chemotherapy. J Clin Oncol 2004; 22(9): 1589–1597.
77. Edelman MJ: An update on the role of epidermal growth factor receptor inhibitors in non-small cell lung cancer. Semin Oncol 2005; 32(6 Suppl 10): S3–S8.

78. Fukuoka M, Yano S, et al: Multi-institutional randomized phase II trial of gefitinib for previously treated patients with advanced non-small-cell lung cancer (The IDEAL 1 Trial) [corrected]. J Clin Oncol 2003; 21(12): 2237–2246.

79. Giaccone G, Herbst R, et al: Gefitinib in combination with gemcitabine and cisplatin in advanced NSCLC: a phase III trial – INTACT 1. J Clin Oncol 2004; 22: 777–784.

80. Herbst R, Giaccone G, et al: Gefitinib in combination with paclitaxel and carboplatin in advanced NSCLC: a phase III trial – INTACT 2. J Clin Oncol 2004; 22: 785–794.

81. Herbst RS, Prager D, et al: TRIBUTE: a phase III trial of erlotinib hydrochloride (OSI-774) combined with carboplatin and pacilitaxel chemotherapy in advanced non-small-cell lung cancer. J Clin Oncol 2005; 23: 5892–5899.

82. Gatzemeier U, Pluzanska A, et al: Results of a phase III trial of erlotinib (OSI-774) combined with cisplatin and gemcitabine (GC) chemotherapy in advanced non-small-cell lung cancer (NSCLC). Proc Am Assoc Clin Oncol 2004; 23: abstr 617.

83. Kris MG, Natale RB, et al: Efficacy of gefitinib, an inhibitor of the epidermal growth factor receptor tyrosine kinase, in symptomatic patients with non-small cell lung cancer: a randomized trial. JAMA 2003; 290: 2149–2158.

84. Shepherd FA, Rodrigues Pereira J, et al: Erlotinib in previously treated non-small-cell lung cancer. N Engl J Med 2005; 353(2): 123–132.

85. Thatcher N, Chang A, et al: Gefitinib plus best supportive care in previously treated patients with refractory advanced non-small-cell lung cancer: Results from a randomised, placebo-controlled, multicentre study (Iressa Survival Evaluation in Lung Cancer). Lancet 2005; 366: 1527–1537.

86. Blackhall F, Ranson M, Thatcher N: Where next for gefitinib in patients with lung cancer? Lancet Oncol 2006; 7; 499–507.

87. Tsao MS, Sakurada A, et al: Erlotinib in lung cancer – molecular and clinical predictors of outcome. N Engl J Med 2005; 353(2): 133–144.

88. Lynch TJ, Bell DW, et al: Activating mutations in the epidermal growth factor receptor underlying responsiveness of non-small-cell lung cancer to gefitinib. N Engl J Med 2004; 350(21): 2129–2139.

89. Paez JG, Janne PA, et al: EGFR mutations in lung cancer: correlation with clinical response to gefitinib therapy. Science 2004; 304(5676): 1497–1500.

90. Hirsch F, Varella-Garcia M, et al: Molecular predictors of outcome with gefitinib in a phase III placebo controlled study in advanced NSCLC. J Clin Oncol 2006; 24(31): 5034–5042.

91. Rocha Lima CM, Herndon JE 2nd, et al: Therapy choices among older patients with lung carcinoma: An evaluation of two trials of the Cancer and Leukemia Group B. Cancer 2002; 94(1): 181–187.

92. Langer CJ, Manola J, et al: Cisplatin-based therapy for elderly patients with advanced non-small-cell lung cancer: implications of Eastern Cooperative Oncology Group 5592, a randomized trial. J Natl Cancer Inst 2002; 94(3): 173–181.

93. Elderly Lung Cancer Vinorelbine Italian Study (ELVIS) Group: Effects of vinorelbine on quality of life and survival of elderly patients with advanced non-small-cell lung cancer. J Natl Cancer Inst 1999; 91: 66–72.

94. Gridelli C, Perrone F, et al: Chemotherapy for elderly patients with advanced non-small-cell lung cancer: The Multicentre Italian Lung Cancer in the Elderly Study (MILES) Phase III randomized trial. J Natl Cancer Inst 2003; 95: 362–372.

95. Sweeney C, Zhu J, et al: Outcome of patients with a performance status of 2 in Eastern Cooperative Group Study EI 1594. Cancer 2001; 92: 2639–2647.
96. Smit E, van Meerbeeck J, et al: Three arm randomized study of two cisplatin based regimens and paclitaxel plus gemcitabine in advanced NSCLC. J Clin Oncol 2003; 21: 3207–3213.
97. Kosmidis P, Mylonakis N, et al: Paclitaxel plus carboplatin versus gemcitabine plus paclitaxel in advanced NSCLC. J Clin Oncol 2002; 20: 3578–3585.
98. Shepherd FA, Ginsberg RJ, et al: Surgical treatment for limited small-cell lung cancer. The University of Toronto Lung Oncology Group experience. J Thorac Cardiovasc Surg 1991; 101(3): 385–393.
99. Szczesny TJ, Szczesna A, Shepherd FA, Ginsberg RJ: Surgical treatment of small cell lung cancer. Semin Oncol 2003; 30(1): 47–56.
100. Jackman DM, Johnson BE: Small-cell lung cancer. Lancet 2005; 366(9494): 1385–1396.
101. Fukuoka M, Furuse K, et al: Randomized trial of cyclophosphamide, doxorubicin, and vincristine versus cisplatin and etoposide versus alternation of these regimens in small-cell lung cancer. J Natl Cancer Inst 1991; 83(12): 855–861.
102. Sundstrom S, Bremnes RM, et al: Cisplatin and etoposide regimen is superior to cyclophosphamide, epirubicin, and vincristine regimen in small-cell lung cancer: Results from a randomized phase III trial with 5 years' follow-up. J Clin Oncol 2002; 20(24): 4665–4672.
103. Jänne P, Freidlin B, et al. Twenty-five years of clinical research for patients with limited stage small cell lung carcinoma in America. Cancer 2002; 95(7): 1528–1538.
104. Chute JP, Chen T, et al: Twenty years of phase III trials for patients with extensive-stage small cell lung cancer perceptible progress. J Clin Oncol 1999; 17: 1794–1801.
105. Pujol JL, Carestia L, Daures J: Is there a case for cisplatin in the treatment of small cell lung cancer: A meta-analysis of randomised trials of a cisplatin containing regimen versus a regimen not containing this alkylating agent. Br J Cancer 2000; 83(1): 8–15.
106. Lorigan P, Woll P, et al: Randomized phase III trial of dose-dense chemotherapy supported by whole-blood haematopoietic progenitors in better-prognosis small cell lung cancer. J Nat Cancer Institute 2005; 97(9): 666–674.
107. James LE, Gower N, et al: A randomised trial of low-dose/high frequency chemotherapy as palliative treatment of poor-prognosis small cell lung cancer. Br J Cancer 1996; 73: 1563–1568.
108. Murray N, Grafton C, et al: Abbreviated treatment for elderly, infirm or non-compliant patients with limited-stage small cell lung cancer. J Clin Oncol 1998; 16(10): 3323–3328.
109. Westeel V, Murray N, et al: New combination of old drugs for elderly patients with small cell lung cancer: a phase II study of the PAVE regimen. J Clin Oncol 1998; 16: 1940–1944.
110. Earl H, Rudd R, et al: Randomised trial of planned versus as required chemotherapy in small cell lung cancer: a Cancer Research Campaign trial. Br J Cancer 1991; 64(3): 566–572.
111. Berghmans T, Paesmans M, et al: A meta-analysis of the role of etoposide and cisplatin in small cell lung cancer with a methodology assessment. Eur J Cancer 1999; 35(S248).

112. Noda K, Nishiwaki Y, Kawahara M, et al: Irinotecan plus cisplatin compared with etoposide plus cisplatin for extensive small cell lung cancer. N Engl J Med 2002; 346: 85–91.

113. Hanna N, Bunn P, et al: Randomized phase III trial comparing irinotecan/cisplatin with etoposide /cisplatin in patients with previously untreated extensive stage SCLC. J Clin Oncol 2006; 24: 2038–2043.

114. Medical Research Council Lung Cancer Working Party. Randomised trial of four drugs versus less intensive two-drug chemotherapy in the palliative treatment of patients with small cell lung cancer and poor prognosis. Br J Cancer. 1996; 74(6): 997.

115. Medical Research Council Lung Cancer Working Party. Comparison of oral etoposide and standard intravenous multi-drug chemotherapy for small cell lung cancer: multicentre randomised trial. Lancet 1996; 348: 563–566.

116. Souhami R, Spiro S, et al: Five day oral etoposide for advanced small cell lung cancer: randomised comparison with intravenous chemotherapy. JNCI 1997; 89: 577–580.

117. White S, Lorigan P, et al: Randomised phase II study of cyclophosphamide, doxorubicin and vincristine compared with single agent carboplatin in patients with poor prognosis small cell lung cancer. Cancer 2001; 92(3): 601–608.

118. O'Brien ME, Ciuleanu TE, et al: Phase II trial comparing supportive care alone with supportive care with oral topotecan in patients with relapsed small-cell lung cancer. J Clin Oncol 2006; 24: 5441–5447.

119. von Pawel J, Schiller J, et al: Topotecan versus cyclophosphamide, vincristine doxorubicin for the treatment of relapsed SCLC. J Clin Oncol 1999; 17: 658–667.

120. von Pawel J, Gatzemeier U, et al: Phase II comparator study of oral versus intravenous topotecan in patients with chemosensitive small-cell lung cancer. J Clin Oncol 2001; 19(16): 1743–1749.

121. Eckardt JR, von Pawel J, et al: Single agent oral topotecan versus intravenous topotecan in patients with chemosensitive small cell lung cancer. Proc Am Soc Clin Oncol 22: 2003; (abstr 2488).

122. Board R, Thatcher N, Lorigan P. New treatments for small cell lung cancer – a time for cautious optimism. Drugs 2006; 66 (15): 1919–1931.

123. Perez C, Einhorn R, et al: Randomised trial of radiotherapy to the thorax in limited small cell carcinoma of the lung treated with multiagent chemotherapy and elective brain irradiation: A preliminary report. J Clin Oncol 1984; 2: 1200–1208.

124. Perry M, Eaton WC, et al: Chemotherapy with or without radiation therapy in limited stage small cell lung cancer. N Engl J Med 1987; 316: 912–918.

125. Bunn PA, Lichter AS, et al. Chemotherapy alone or chemotherapy with chest radiation therapy in limited-stage small-cell lung cancer. Ann Int Med 1987; 106: 655–662.

126. Pignon JP, Arriagada R, et al: A meta-analysis of thoracic radiotherapy for small-cell lung cancer. N Engl J Med 1992; 327: 1618–1622.

127. Warde P, Payne D: Does thoracic irradiation improve survival and local control in in limited-stage small-cell lung cancer. J Clin Oncol 1992; 10: 890–895.

128. Turrisi AT, Kim K, et al: Twice daily compared to once-daily thoracic radiotherapy in limited-stage small-cell lung cancer treated concurrently with cisplatin and etoposide. N Engl J Med 1999; 340: 265–271.

129. Takada M, Fukuoka M, et al: Phase III study of concurrent versus sequential thoracic radiotherapy in combination with cisplatin and etoposide for limited-stage small-cell lung cancer: results of the Japan Clinical Oncology Group Study 9104. J Clin Oncol 2002; 20(14): 3054–3060.

130. Jeremic B, Shibamoto Y, et al: Initial versus delayed accelerated hyperfractionated radiation therapy and concurrent chemotherapy in limited small-cell lung cancer: A randomized study. J Clin Oncol 1997; 15(3): 893–900.

131. Murray N, Coy P, et al: Importance of timing for thoracic irradiation in the combined modality treatment of limited-stage small-cell lung cancer. The National Cancer Institute of Canada Clinical Trials Group. J Clin Oncol 1993; 11(2): 336–344.

132. De Ruysscher D, Pijls-Johannesma M, et al: Systematic review and meta-analysis of randomized, controlled trials of the timing of chest radiotherapy in patients with limited-stage, small-cell lung cancer. Ann Oncol 2006; 17(4): 543–552.

133. Fried B, Morris D, Hensing T, et al: Systematic review evaluating the timing of thoracic radiation therapy in combined modality therapy for limited stage small-cell lung cancer. J Clin Oncol 2004; 22: 4785–4793.

134. de Ruysscher D, Pijls-Johannesma M, Bentzen S, et al: Time between the first day of chemotherapy and the last day of chest radiation is the most important predictor of survival in limited-disease small-cell lung cancer. J Clin Oncol 2006; 24(7): 1057–1063.

135. Aupérin A, Arriagada R, Pignon JP, et al: Prophylactic cranial irradiation for patients with small-cell lung cancer in complete remission. Prophylactic Cranial Irradiation Overview Collaborative Group. N Engl J Med 1999; 341(7): 476–484.

136. Komaki R, Meyers CA, Shin DM, et al: Evaluation of cognitive function in patients with limited small cell lung cancer prior to and shortly following prophylactic cranial irradiation. Int J Radiat Oncol Biol Phys 1995; 33(1): 179–182.

Systemic and mucocutaneous reactions to chemotherapy

5

Joseph P. Eder and Arthur T. Skarin

Cancer chemotherapy is a major component of cancer therapy, along with surgery and radiation. Cancer chemotherapy agents differ from most drugs in that it is intentionally cytotoxic to human cells. This aspect of cancer chemotherapeutic agents produces a narrow therapeutic index (desired vs. undesired effects) for most, but not all, agents in this class. The target of cancer chemotherapeutic agents is the proliferating cancer cell. While many normal tissues are non-proliferating, some are proliferating and toxicity of this class tends to preferentially overlap proliferating tissues – haematopoietic, gastrointestinal mucosa and skin. In addition, each agent often has specific organ toxicity related to its chemical class or unique mechanism of action.

The major groups of cancer chemotherapeutic agents are the direct-acting alkylating agents, the indirect-acting anthracyclines and topoisomerase inhibitors, the antimetabolites, the tubulin-binding agents, hormones, receptor-targeted agents and a class of miscellaneous agents. Despite the disparate nature of this broad class of agents, some generalizations about the effects of chemotherapy are still possible. For more information readers are referred to detailed reports.[1,2]

ACUTE HYPERSENSITIVITY REACTIONS

Acute hypersensitivity can occur with any drug. However, several cancer chemotherapeutic agents are derived from hydrophobic plant chemicals and must be solubilized with agents with a marked propensity for causing acute hypersensitivity reactions, especially histamine-mediated anaphylactic reactions, such as the Cremophor used with paclitaxel. Docetaxel has a lower incidence of this complication.

The incidence of severe hypersensitivity reactions with paclitaxel may be up to 25% without ancillary measures. With antihistamine H1 and H2 blockade and corticosteroids, the incidence falls to 2–3%. Hypersensitivity reactions occur in up to 40% of patients receiving single agent 1-asparaginase but only 20% when administered in combination therapy with glucocorticoids and 6-mercaptopurine, perhaps as a result of immunosuppression. The hypersensitivity usually occurs after several doses and in successive cycles. The reaction may be only urticaria (see Figure 5.1) but may be severe with laryngospasm or, rarely, serum sickness. Fatal reactions occur <1% of the time. Changing the source of enzyme is the appropriate initial step. Two other proteins in

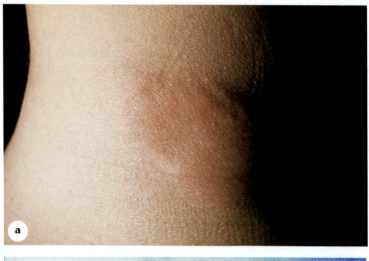

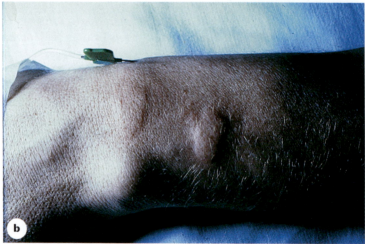

Fig. 5.1 Acute hypersensitivity reactions. Urticaria, with giant localized hives, occurred (**a**) in a 40-year-old man within a few minutes of receiving intravenous 5-fluorouracil and (**b**) in the lower arm of a 50-year-old man after receiving adriamycin. The urticaria was self-limiting in both patients.

clinical use, rituximab and traztuzumab, have a similar incidence of hypersensitivity reactions.

Certain drugs such as etoposide are associated with a greater incidence of reactions but most are not true hypersensitivity reactions. The Tween diluant in the clinical etoposide formulation produces hypotension, rash and back pain. The platinum compounds carboplatin and cisplatin are associated with hypersensitivity reactions, particularly on subsequent cycles – most of these reactions are severe (75%).[3] Hypersensitivity to platinum and related compounds is actually quite frequent, up to 14% in industrial workers, so such reactions in patients receiving these agents parenterally should not be surprising and is often unappreciated in combination chemotherapy regimens, such as with taxanes, and may be equally suppressed by the prophylactic regimens employed.[4] Liposomal encapsulated anthracyclines are associated with an increased incidence of hypersensitivity compared with the parent drugs. Like the reaction to Cremophor EL and radiocontrast agents, the reaction is a "complement activation pseudoallergy".[5] Up to 45% of cancer patients show activation of the classical, alternative or both complement pathways, although the incidence of clinical reactions is about 20%.

Monoclonal antibodies such as trastuzumab, rituximab, bevacizumab, and cetuximab have had enormous impact on cancer therapeutics. Monoclonal antibodies may be chimeric (a murine Fab binding site but human amino acid sequences elsewhere) or fully human. Allergic or hypersensitivity reactions are more frequent with chimeric proteins such as cetuximab (1–5% clinically significant) and are treated with antihistamines and steroids plus slowing of the infusion. L-Asparaginase is a bacterial protein that frequently results in hypersensitivity reactions. These reactions are more frequent with interrupted schedules and with subsequent re-challenge. Changing the source from *Escherichia coli* to *Erwinia* is one accepted strategem if immunosuppression does not work.

ALOPECIA

Many antineoplastic drugs can produce marked hair loss (see Figure 5.2). This includes not only scalp hair but also facial, axillary, pubic and all body hair. The germinating hair follicle has an approximately 24-hour doubling time. Cancer chemotherapy agents preferentially affect actively growing (anagen) hairs. The interruption of mitosis produces a structurally weakened hair prone to fracture easily from minimal trauma such as brushing. Since 80–90% of scalp hairs are in anagen phase, the degree

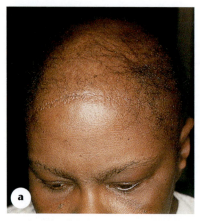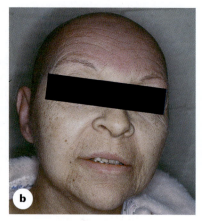

Fig. 5.2 Alopecia. (**a**) Near-total alopecia in a 38-year-old woman receiving cyclophosphamide and adriamycin. Note the loss of eyebrow and eyelid hair. (**b**) Total alopecia developed in this 64-year-old woman due to chemotherapy and cranial irradiation for brain metastases. The duration of alopecia after both treatment modalities may be many months or even permanent in some patients. In this woman, the scalp oedema and erythema are related to an allergic cutaneous reaction from diphenyl hydantoin.

of hair loss can be substantial. Hair loss, while often emotionally difficult for patients, is reversible, although hair may regrow more curly and of a slightly different colour.

STOMATITIS/MUCOSITIS

The oral complications of cancer chemotherapy are many and frequently severe. The disruption of the protective mucosal barrier serves as a portal of entry for pathogens which, especially when combined with chemotherapy-induced neutropenia, predisposes to local infection and systemic sepsis. Once established, these infections may be difficult to eradicate in immunocompromised patients. The most common infectious organisms are *Candida albicans*, herpes simplex virus, β-haemolytic streptococci, staphylococci, opportunistic Gram-negative bacteria and mouth anaerobes.

Several agents of the antimetabolite class of cancer chemotherapeutic agents, especially those that target pyrimidine biosynthesis such as methotrexate, 5-fluorouracil (5-FU) and cytosine arabinoside, and the anthracycline agents, such as doxorubicin and daunorubicin, are particularly toxic to the mucosal epithelium (see Figure 5.3). These agents

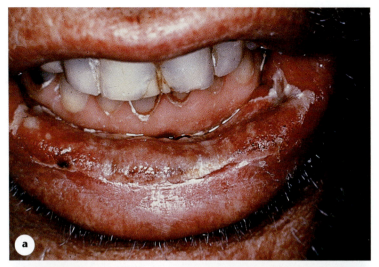

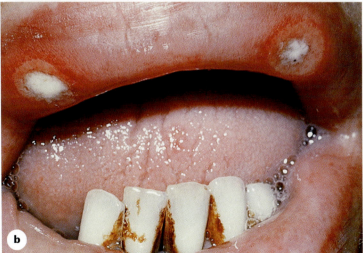

Fig. 5.3 Stomatitis and mucositis. (**a**) Marked stomatitis in a patient receiving methotrexate. (**b**) Aphthous stomatitis related to severe granulocytopenia after chemotherapy. The ulcers may be due to herpes simplex or other infection.

have a marked capacity to produce more severe injury in irradiated tissues, even if the radiation is temporally remote. These agents produce marked ulceration and erosion of the mucosa. These lesions occur initially on those mucosal surfaces that abrade the teeth and gums, such as the sides of the tongue, the vermillion border of the lower lip and the

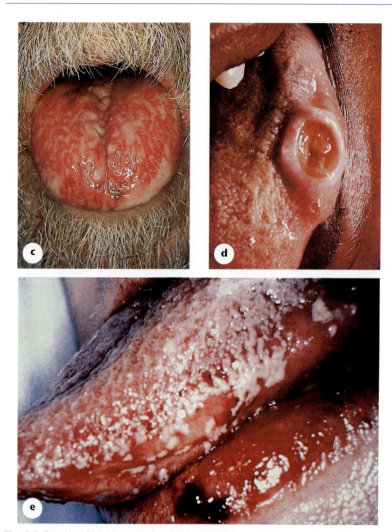

Fig. 5.3 *Continued* (**c**) Mucositis in a patient receiving combination chemotherapy for head and neck cancer. (**d**) Marked ulcer of the tongue in a 32-year-old man receiving induction chemotherapy for acute leukaemia. (**e**) Mucositis of the tongue due to monilia infection (thrush) in a patient receiving corticosteroids for brain metastases.

buccal mucosa. More advanced mucosal injury may occur on the hard and soft palate and the posterior oropharynx. These ulcerations cannot often be distinguished from those caused by infectious organisms. Appropriate tests must be performed to exclude viral, fungal and bacterial causes or superinfection.

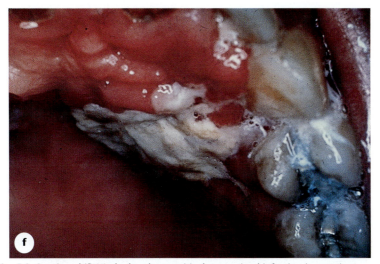

Fig. 5.3 *Continued* **(f)** Marked oral mucositis due to mixed infection in a patient receiving chemotherapy for acute leukaemia.

In addition to the risk of infection, the resultant pain makes patients unable to maintain adequate nutrition and hydration. This may compromise the capacity to complete a course of chemotherapy and require prolonged administration of parenteral fluids and even parenteral nutrition.

DERMATITIS, SKIN RASHES AND HYPERPIGMENTATION

Superficial manifestations of cancer chemotherapy agents are noted frequently by patients, although they are considered significant much less often by clinicians. The cosmetic changes may be disturbing to patients without requiring discontinuation of therapy.

Of the direct-acting alkylating agents, busulfan has been associated with a wide variety of specific and non-specific cutaneous changes. Diffuse hyperpigmentation has been noted (see Figure 5.4), which resolves with discontinuation of therapy. Systemic mechlorethamine (nitrogen mustard) has no cutaneous toxicity. However, when applied topically for cutaneous T-cell lymphomas, telangiectasias, hyperpigmentation and allergic contact dermatitis may occur. The development of more effective, safer alternative agents has rendered busulfan and mechlorethamine to essentially historical interest only or narrow

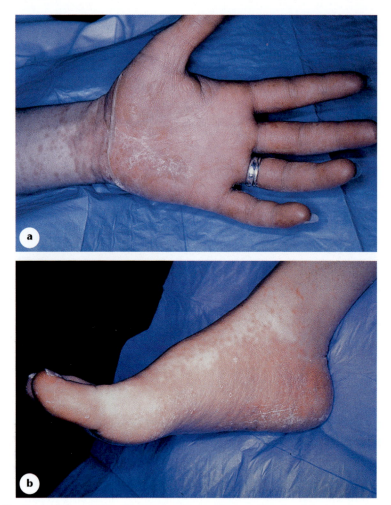

Fig. 5.4 (a,b) Dermatitis, skin rashes and hyperpigmentation: hand–foot syndrome related to 5-fluorouracil chemotherapy in metastatic colon cancer. Note the erythema, oedema, rash and early skin desquamation. Severe pain is associated with this toxic reaction.

indications (busulfan in allogeneic bone marrow transplant for haematological malignancies). Cyclophosphamide, ifosfamide and melphalan produce hyperpigmentation of nails, teeth, gingiva and skin.

The antimetabolites methotrexate and 5-FU are frequently associated with cutaneous reactions. In contrast, the purine antimetabolites

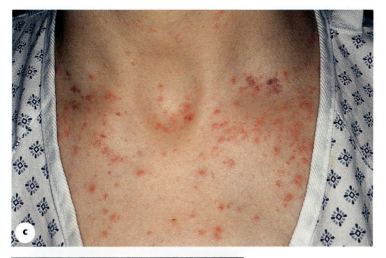

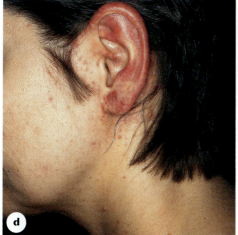

Fig. 5.4 *Continued* **(c,d)** Skin reaction to Ara-C. Note the erythematous macular rash on the chest and diffuse erythema and oedema of the ears in this 22-year-old woman receiving Ara-C for acute leukaemia.

6-mercaptopurine, 6-thioguanine, cladribine, fludarabine and pento-statin are devoid of cutaneous toxicity. Methotrexate, a folate antago-nist, may cause reactivation of ultraviolet burns when given in close proximity to previous sun exposure. This is not prevented by leucov-orin, a reduced folate that prevents the myelosuppression and stom-

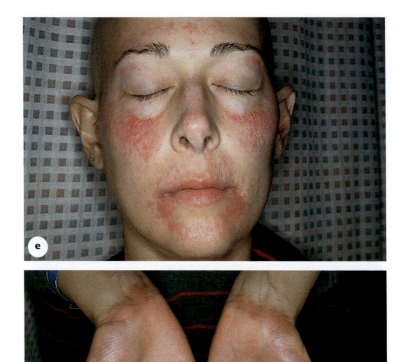

Fig. 5.4 *Continued* **(e,f)** Skin reaction to docetaxel. Note periorbital and malar flush along with erythema and oedema of the palms in this patient.

atitis of high doses of methotrexate. Methotrexate should be given more than a week after a significant solar burn. It may cause stomatitis and cutaneous ulcerations at high dose, despite the use of leucovorin. Extensive epidermal necrolysis may occur and be fatal. Multiple areas of vesiculation and erosion over pressure areas have been noticed.

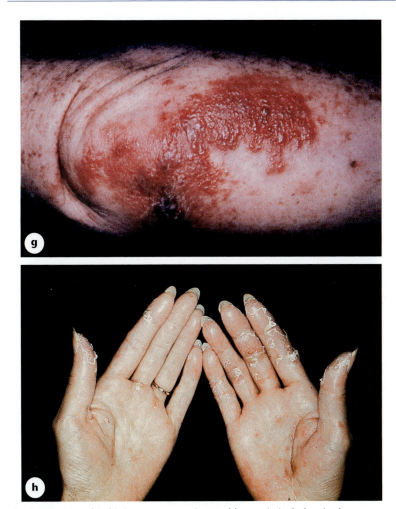

Fig. 5.4 *Continued* (**g,h**) Cutaneous reactions to bleomycin include raised, erythematous and pruritic lesions around pressure points, especially the elbows (**g**), as well as desquamation of skin (**h**).

5-FU is an antimetabolite with steric properties similar to uracil. Like methotrexate, 5-FU produces increased sensitivity to ultraviolet-induced toxic reactions in a large number of patients, over 35% in one study. Enhanced sunburn erythema and increased posterythema hyper-pigmentation characterize these reactions. A hyperpigmentation reaction over the veins in which the drug is administered may occur. This is

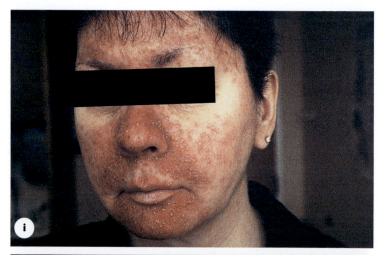

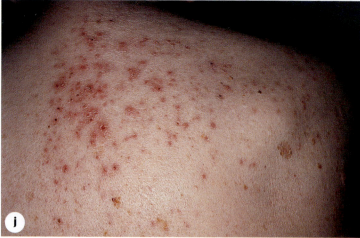

Fig. 5.4 *Continued* (**i,j**) Acneiform skin lesions occur in patients on gefitinib, especially on the face (**i**), chest and back (**j**). These rashes may regress when the drug is temporarily withheld or the dose is lowered. Similar skin reactions occur after actinomycin D and corticosteroids.

probably hyperpigmentation secondary to chemical phlebitis due to chemotherapeutic agents in the superficial venous system. Nail and generalized skin hyperpigmentation have been reported with 5-FU. Occasionally, acute inflammation of existing actinic keratosis is seen in patients receiving 5-FU. This differs from a drug reaction in that it occurs in discrete inflamed regions only in sun-exposed areas, not in a

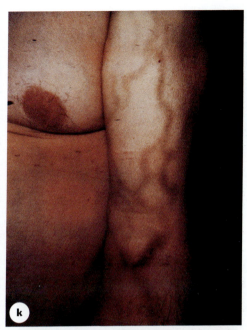

Fig. 5.4 *Continued* (k) Hyperpigmentation of the skin along veins occurs after the use of many chemotherapeutic agents, including Navelbine, actinomycin D and 5-fluorouracil infusion, as in this patient. In many cases, the veins become sclerotic due to thrombophlebitis. (l–n) Hyperpigmentation of the skin after 5-fluorouracil (l), *Continued*

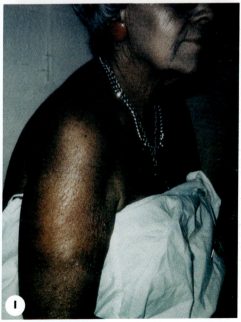

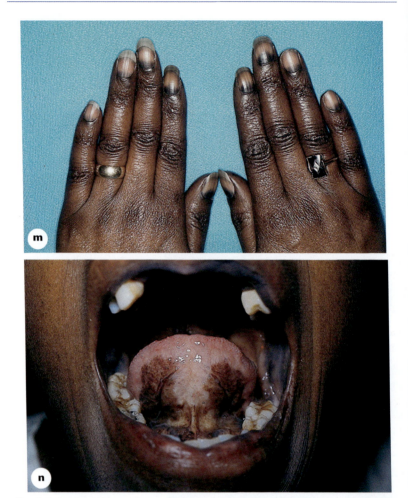

Fig. 5.4 *Continued* Hyperpigmentation of the skin occurs after adriamycin and other drugs (**m**), while increased pigment in the mucous membranes (**n**) and nails (**m**) is mainly related to adriamycin. (Also see Fig. 5.6b).

generalized distribution. The end result is usually the disappearance of the actinic keratosis as a result of an inflammatory infiltration into the atypical epidermis and resultant removal of atypical cells.

When 5-FU is given by intravenous continuous infusion, the most common dose-limiting toxicity is erythromalagia, the so-called hand–foot syndrome (see Figure 5.4). The hands and feet become red, oedematous and often painful. The skin often peels afterwards. The nails become dry and brittle and develop linear cracks. This may occur at doses less than those that produce the hand–foot syndrome. Other drugs that can result in this syndrome include new, targeted therapy drugs, such as sorafenib and sunitinib, which have multiple targets including vascular endothelial growth factor (VEGF) receptor. A similar reaction occurs with 5-FU or 5-FU prodrugs administered orally on a daily schedule. Capecitabine, an oral prodrug that is eventually converted to 5-FU intracellularly, produces erythromalagia as its most common toxicity. Interestingly, oral 5-FU does not produce this syndrome when combined with enyluracil, an irreversible inhibitor of dihydropyrimidine dehydrogenase, the major enzyme in 5-FU catabolism.

High doses of cytosine arabinoside may produce ocular toxicity through an ulcerating keratoconjunctivitis. This may be prevented by the prophylactic administration of steroid eyedrops. Excessive lacrimation may be noted with 5-FU therapy due to lacrimal duct stenosis. This is corrected by surgical dilatation of the duct.

The indirect acting anticancer drugs may produce superficial cutaneous toxicity. The anthracyclines doxorubicin, daunorubicin, epirubicin and idarubicin produce complete alopecia. Radiation recall reactions are frequent, even when the two modalities are separated by years. Skin, nail and mucous membrane hyperpigmentation may be striking; these may be localized or general. Hyperpigmentation of the hands, feet and face may occur in patients of African descent. Liposomal anthracyclines, such as Doxil (doxorubicin) and Daunosome (daunorubicin), may produce a severe erythromayalagia with palmar and plantar erythema and desquamation similar to 5-FU. Actinomycin D produces a characteristic skin eruption in many patients. Beginning 3–5 days after drug administration, patients develop facial erythema followed by papules, pustules and plugged follicles similar to the open comedones of acne. This eruption is benign, self-limited and not a reason to stop therapy. A similar acneiform skin rash occurs in patients taking the new oral epidermal growth factor receptor inhibitors such as gefitinib and erlotinib (see Figure 5.4). In most patients the rash is mild and may regress with continued treatment. When severe, the skin lesions will rapidly regress with discontinuation of the drug. Topical steroids and antibiotics may be indicated.

Bleomycin is actually a mixture of peptides isolated from *Streptomyces verticullus*. Its most common toxic effects involve the lungs and skin because of high concentrations in these organs due to the deficiency of the catabolic enzyme bleomycin hydrolase in these tissues. Cutaneous toxicity occurs in the majority of patients treated with bleomycin doses in excess of 200 mg. Bleomycin causes a morbilliform eruption 30 minutes to 3 hours after administration in approximately 10% of patients (see Figure 5.4). It most likely represents a transient hypersensitivity response (it may be accompanied by fever). Linear or "flagellate" hyperpigmentation may occur on the trunk. This may likewise represent postinflammatory hyperpigmentation. Bleomycin may cause a scleroderma-like eruption of the skin. Infiltrative plaques, nodules and linear bands of the hands have been described. Pathological findings include dermal sclerosis and appendage entrapment similar to that seen in scleroderma. These changes are reversible when the drug is stopped.

Etoposide has relatively few cutaneous manifestations at standard doses (<600 mg/m^2). At higher doses (1800–4200 mg/m^2), a generalized pruritic, erythematous, maculopapular rash occurs in approximately 25% of patients. The most severe toxicity occurs at the highest doses. In these patients, an intense, well-defined palmar erythema develops. Affected areas become oedematous, red and painful. Bullus formation and desquamation follow. The severity of the reaction is related to dose. A short course (3–5 days) of corticosteroids controls the symptoms.

Sorafenib and a related drug, sunitinib malate, are oral multi-targeted receptor tyrosine kinase inhibitors that block signal transduction through the *raf* kinases, vascular endothelial growth factor receptor 2 (VEGFR2) and the platelet-derived growth factor receptors. At the recommended dose there is a 33% incidence of skin rashes or desquamation, 27% incidence of hand–foot syndome and 22% incidence of alopecia (all grades of severity).[6]

Cutaneous rashes are the most common toxicities encountered with gefitinib and erlotinib. The chimeric monoclonal antibodies cetuximab and panitumumab are associated with dermatological toxicity. The severity and extent of the skin changes, including dry skin, desquamation, erythema, nail changes and acneiform eruptions varies from report to report and no consistent grading system for incidence and severity is universally agreed upon. There is neutrophil and macrophage infiltration of the dermis and hair follicles, with thinning of the epidermis and stratum corneum. The incidence and severity is dose-dependent. Certain epidermal growth factor receptor polymorphisms increase the incidence of developing a rash. For erlotinib, cetuximab and panitumumab, several studies support a positive correlation between development of a rash and response, and rash and survival.[7] Management is usually supportive with creams, including 1% clindamycin, 5% benzoyl peroxide and systemic antibiotics when there is evidence of infection, including tetracycline and amoxicillin/clavulinate. These should be used only when necessary.

SKIN ULCERATION AND EXTRAVASATION

Vesicant reactions from extravasated cancer chemotherapeutic agents are one of the most debilitating complications seen with cancer therapy (see Figure 5.5). The anthracyclines, especially doxorubicin, are particularly noted for an intense inflammatory chemical cellulitis caused by

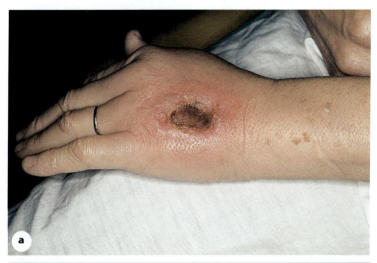

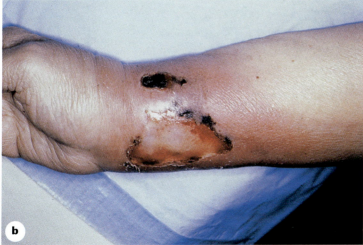

Fig. 5.5 (a–d) Extravasation of drugs and skin ulcers occurs with vesicant drugs. Acute changes with adriamycin (**a,b**)

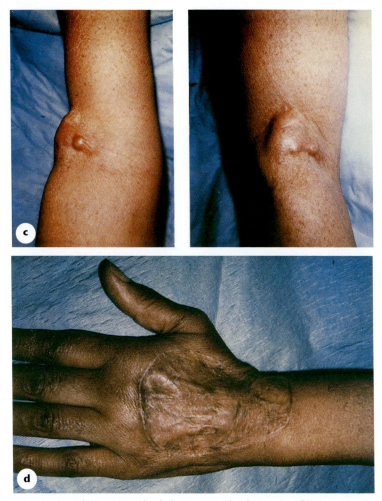

Fig. 5.5 *Continued* (**c**) Chronic healed scarring with adriamycin, (**d**) mitomycin-C. Other drugs include actinomycin D, vincristine and Navelbine. Immediate medical attention is necessary and sometimes skin grafts are required (see text).

subcutaneous extravasation. This results in ulceration and necrosis of affected tissue. No local measures have proven unequivocally helpful once the accident has occurred. Doxorubicin should be stopped immediately but the intravenous line left in place. Dilution of doxorubicin with sodium bicarbonate and the local installation of steroids prior to catheter withdrawal are standard measures but their efficacy is uncertain. Rest and warm compresses are recommended. If healing does not proceed well, excision of the affected area and surgical grafting are recommended to avoid excess morbidity. Other agents with vesicant properties include the vinca alkaloids (vincristine, vinblastine, vinorelbine) and actinomycin. General recommendations for the administration of vesicant drugs include the use of veins as far away from the hands and joints as possible and that the intravenous line be able to infuse at a rapid rate and have a good blood return. The use of venous access devices is accepted as appropriate in this situation unless contraindicated on specific clinical grounds.

Generalized skin ulceration is an infrequent, albeit dramatic, occurrence. Mucocutaneous ulcerations are frequently noted with bleomycin. These begin as oedema and erythema over pressure points such as the elbows, knees and fingertips and in intertrigenous areas such as the groin and axillae. These areas then proceed to shallow ulcerations. These ulcerations may also occur in the oral cavity. Biopsy shows epidermal degeneration and necrosis with dermal oedema. Total epidermal necrosis can even be found without any dermal changes. This suggests that the epidermal toxicity is the primary event.

NAIL CHANGES

Banding of the nails is the appearance of linear horizontal depressions in the nails that occur as a result of growth interruptions in the nail germinal cell layer by a cytostatic effect from the administration of cancer chemotherapy agents. These occur in other disease settings and are called Beau's lines (see Figure 5.6). The direct-acting alkylating agents cyclophosphamide, ifosfamide and melphalan may also produce hyperpigmentation of nails. The nails may exhibit linear or transverse banding or hyperpigmentation. These changes begin proximally and progress distally and clear, proximally to distally, when the agents are discontinued. Similar effects are seen with the indirect–acting anthracyclines, such as doxorubicin, and bleomycin. The anthracyclines may cause hyperpigmentation of the hyponychia (the soft layer of skin beneath the nail), especially in dark-skinned persons.

Onycholysis is separation of the nail plate from the nail bed (see Figure 5.6). Anthracyclines, anthracenediones and taxanes are the drugs most frequently associated with onycholysis. The combination of these agents is most frequently reported with onycholysis. Most of the reports are associated with docetaxel, either administered weekly or every 3

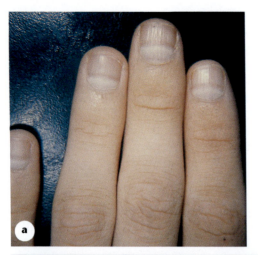

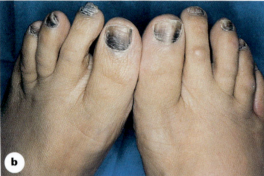

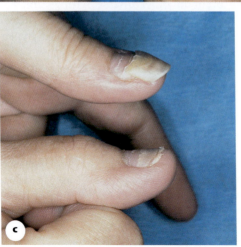

Fig. 5.6 Nail changes are often seen after prolonged chemotherapy. (**a**) Banding of the nails results from growth interruptions in the nail germinal cell layer by the cytostatic effect of chemotherapy. These white bands (called Mee's lines) will grow outward eventually. Beau's lines are transverse grooves across the nail plate due to temporary nail matrix malfunction, seen with chemotherapy or associated with other illnesses (acute coronary or severe febrile episodes). Nail hyperpigmentation occurs occasionally after prolonged use of adriamycin (**b**) especially in people with dark skin. Onycholysis or separation of the nail from its bed is associated with use of adriamycin (**c**), cyclophosphamide and the taxanes.

weeks. These changes occur after hyperpigmentation of the hyponychia, often with hyperkeratosis and splinter haemorrhages. Ultraviolet light may be a facilitating factor. Onycholysis can occur within weeks or months of the initiation of therapy.

RADIATION RECALL

Radiation recall dermatitis is a cutaneous toxicity that develops in patients with prior exposure to therapeutic doses of radiation and subsequent treatment with a cancer chemotherapeutic agent (see Figure 5.7). These reactions occur in the previously irradiated field and not elsewhere. A previous cutaneous reaction at the time of irradiation is not a prerequisite. The onset of symptoms is days to weeks after drug treatment and can occur any time after radiation, even years later. Cutaneous manifestations include erythema with maculopapular eruptions, vesiculation and desquamation. The intensity of the cutaneous response can vary from a mild rash to skin necrosis. Radiation recall reactions in other organs can produce gastrointestinal mucosal inflammation (stomatitis, oesophagitis, enteritis, proctitis), pneumonitis and myocarditis.

An extensive number of anticancer agents have been implicated in radiation recall reactions. The anthracyclines (doxorubicin as an example), bleomycin, dactinomycin, etoposide, the taxanes, vinca alkaloids and antimetabolites (hydroxycarbamide, fluorouracil, methotrexate, gemcitabine) are the most commonly implicated in cutaneous toxicity. In addition, these skin reactions have been seen in association with targeted therapy with drugs such as gefitinib.

Methotrexate and dactinomycin are reported to cause radiation enhancement in the central nervous system (CNS). The antimetabolites doxorubicin, dactinomycin and bleomycin enhance gastrointestinal toxicity from radiation. Cyclophosphamide, taxanes, hydroxycarbamide, doxorubicin, dactinomycin, gemcitabine, cytosine arabinoside and, most importantly, bleomycin exacerbate pulmonary radiation toxicity. Optic toxicity is increased by treatment with fluorouracil and cytosine arabinoside. Radiation lowers the dose of doxorubicin that produces cardiomyopathy.

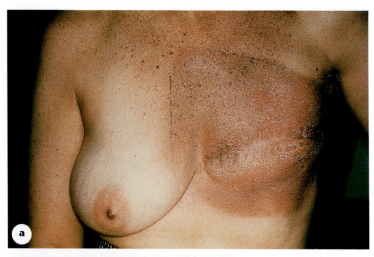

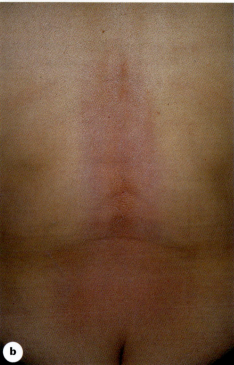

Fig. 5.7 Radiation recall dermatitis may occur in a radiotherapy treatment field after systemic chemotherapy, with development of hyperaemia and then hyperpigmentation in the healing phase (**a**). The patient in (**a**) received adjuvant Alkeran (melphalan) 1 month after postoperative radiation to the chest wall. (**b**) This patient had radiation therapy to the lower spine for bone metastases from breast cancer and developed recall dermatitis 6 months later, when gemcitabine was administered.

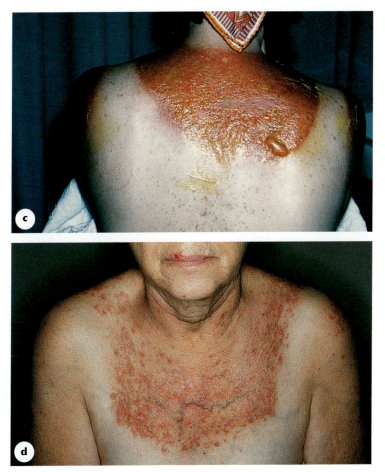

Fig. 5.7 *Continued* (**c**) Chemotherapy can also sensitize the skin to adverse reactions to solar radiation. This young woman developed severe dermatitis in a sun-exposed area while taking methotrexate. (**d**) This patient also developed acute dermatitis in a sun-exposed area while receiving 5-fluorouracil.

ORGAN TOXICITY

CARDIAC AND CARDIOVASCULAR TOXICITY

Cardiotoxicity is a well-recognized consequence of anthracycline use, especially doxorubicin because of its wide spectrum of antineoplastic therapy. This peculiar and potentially lethal problem can be classified as acute or chronic. The acute toxicity is usually asymptomatic arrhythmias, including heart block. Acute myopericarditis occurs at low total doses in an idiosyncratic fashion or at high single doses >110–120 mg/m^2. Fever, pericarditis and congestive heart failure (CHF) are the clinical manifestations. Chronic cardiomyopathy is characterized by progressive myofibrillar damage with each dose, dilatation of sarcoplasmic reticulum, loss of myofibrils and myocardial necrosis/fibrosis. Various syndromes of cardiac toxicity related to antineoplastic agents have been recently reviewed in detail.[8] Imatinib mesylate used commonly in chronic myelogenous leukaemia and gastrointestinal stromal tumours, has been associated with a low incidence of cardiomyopathy syndrome.[9]

A doxorubicin total dose <550 mg/m^2 has a 1–10% occurrence of CHF (daunorubicin 900–1000 mg/m^2), a 40% incidence at 800 mg/m^2 of doxorubicin, and the incidence of CHF approaches 100% at 1 g/m^2. Cardiac function is tested using non-invasive techniques to measure the resting and exercise ejection fraction, including radionuclide ventriculograms and echocardiograms, or invasively by cardiac biopsy. Factors that increase the risk of developing CHF include pre-existing heart disease, hypertension and cardiac radiation therapy. Concomitant dosing with trastuzamab increases the cardiac toxicity of doxorubicin. Cardiac toxicity is a function of *peak* dose level, so continuous infusions or weekly dosing decrease the risk. Desrazoxane, an iron chelator, decreases cardiotoxicity and is approved for use.

Biochemical mechanisms implicated include calcium-mediated damage to the sarcoplasmic reticulum which increases calcium ion (Ca^{++}) release with increased Ca^{++} uptake in mitochondria in preference to ATP. Lipid peroxidations of the sarcoplasmic reticulum, which decrease high Ca^{++} binding sites, and lipid peroxidation due to drug $\cdot$Fe^{3+} complexes with hydroxyl (OH) radical generation may contribute to cardiotoxicity. The heart has no catalase, and anthracyclines decrease glutathione peroxidase activity, which increases the sensitivity of the myocardium to oxidative damage.

Idarubicin and epirubicin have less cardiotoxicity but are still capable of causing cardiotoxicity. High-dose cyclophosphamide, at doses

>60 mg/kg as used in bone marrow transplantation, can cause a haemorrhagic cardiomyopathy. Paclitaxel produces clinically insignificant atrial arrhythmias. Agents that can produce arterial smooth muscle spasm may produce ischaemic myocardial infarction in the absence of fixed coronary vascular disease. These agents include 5-FU, vincristine and vinblastine.

Combination chemotherapy in colorectal cancer with bevacizumab has been associated with an incidence (1–3%) of ischaemic cardiac events above that observed with conventional therapy alone. This increase in cardiovascular events, while of low overall incidence, nonetheless represents about a 3-fold increase.[10]

Sunitinib has a 10% incidence of usually reversible cardiomyopathy. Patients can often be treated with lower doses if and when symptoms resolve.[11]

Hypertension has been recognized as a class effect for agents that target VEGFR2. Hypertension is so common that it serves as a pharmacodynamic endpoint in the early development of agents of this class. Hypertension of a moderate degree (grade 2, recurrent or persistent, symptomatic increase of diastolic blood pressure >200 mmHg or to >150/100 mmHg or requiring monotherapy) or severe degree (grade 3, requiring more than one agent or more intensive therapy) occurs in 10–25% of patients receiving bevacizumab, sorafenib or sunitinib. Patients with pre-existing or borderline hypertension are more susceptible. No specific treatment algorithmn has yet been applied to the management of these patients.

PULMONARY TOXICITY

Bleomycin produces pulmonary toxicity, which is the major problem with subacute or chronic interstitial pneumonitis complicated by late-stage fibrosis (see Figure 5.8). The incidence is 3–5% with doses <450 u/m^2, in patients over 70, with emphysema and after high single doses (>25 u/m^2). The incidence rises to 10% at doses >450 mg/m^2, but can occur at cumulative doses <100 mg. Pulmonary injury can occur during high FiO$_2$ and volume overload during surgery for many years after exposure.

Toxicity results from free radicals produced by an intercalated Fe(II)–bleomycin–O$_2$ complex between DNA strands. Intercalation of drug into the DNA is the first step; then Fe(II) is oxidized and O$_2$ is reduced to oxygen ($^{\bullet}$O$_2$) or hydroxyl radicals $^{\bullet}$OH. DNA cleavage occurs after the activated bleomycin complex is assembled. Strand breakage absolutely requires O$_2$, which is converted to O$_{2-}$ and $^{\bullet}$OH, and peroxidation products of DNA (and protein) are formed. Free radical scavengers and superoxide dismutase inhibit DNA breakage. Bleomycin is hydrolyzed by

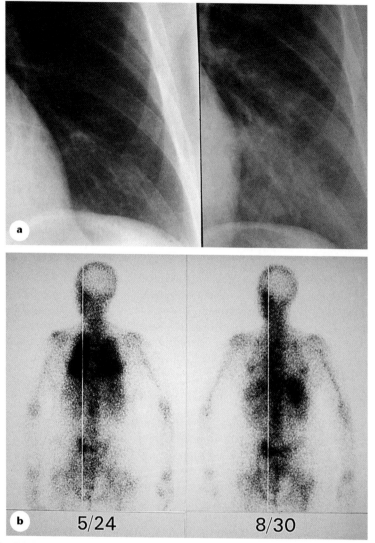

Fig. 5.8 Organ toxicity. Non-mucocutaneous toxicity of chemotherapeutic agents is covered in the text. The lung may be affected by several agents including bleomycin. (a) The earliest radiographic changes are linear infiltrates in the lower lung fields. (b) Gallium-67 uptake is quite striking but is reversible, as this serial study demonstrates.

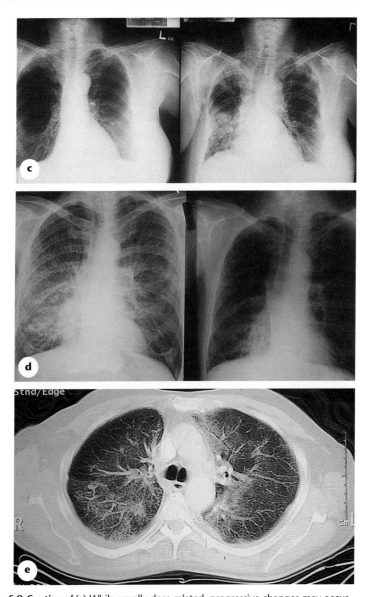

Fig. 5.8 *Continued* (c) While usually dose related, progressive changes may occur resulting in fibrosis and pulmonary insufficiency. Other drugs such as alkylating agents and high-dose methotrexate may result in diffuse infiltrates (**d**), which were reversible 4 months later. (**e**) In this patient several courses of gemcitabine resulted in acute dyspnoea and decreased oxygen saturation. Evaluation with lung biopsy and other studies showed no evidence of infection, pulmonary emboli or other diagnosable disease. Use of prednisone led to rapid improvement and regression of the interstitial infiltrates.

bleomycin hydrolase, a cysteine present in normal and malignant cells but decreased in lung and skin.

Busulfan, mitomycin C and carmustine are direct-acting alkylating agents that can cause chronic interstitial pneumonitis and fibrosing alveolitis. This chronic fibrosis produces the clinical picture of progressive, often fatal, restrictive lung disease. The symptoms occur insidiously, often after prolonged therapy. The chronic use of busulfan for the treatment of chronic myelogenous leukaemia is now a historical footnote but carmustine remains the mainstay of treatment for glioblastoma and anaplastic astrocytomas. Cyclophosphamide has been implicated in chronic pulmonary toxicity but rarely as a single agent, more often after radiation.

The antimetabolite methotrexate may produce an acute eosinophilic pneumonitis, which represents an allergic reaction. Cytosine arabinoside and gemcitabine (2',2'-difluoro-2'-deoxycytidine) may also cause an acute pneumonitis, which may be fatal if unrecognized. In these circumstances, withdrawal of the offending agent, supportive care and corticosteroids may prevent a fatal outcome.[12] Some of the reported pulmonary syndromes associated with chemotherapy drugs are noted in Table 5.1.

Table 5.1 Pulmonary syndromes associated with specific cancer chemotherapy drugs

Syndrome	Associated cancer chemotherapy drugs
Pulmonary capillary leak	Interleukin-2, recombinant tumour necrosis factor alpha, cytarabine, mitomycin
Asthma	Interleukin-2, vinca alkaloids plus mitomycin
Bronchiolitis obliterans organizing pneumonia	Bleomycin, cyclophosphamide, methotrexate, mitomycin
Hypersensitivity pneumonitis	Busulfan, bleomycin, etoposide, methotrexate, mitomycin, procarbazine
Interstitial pneumonia/fibrosis	Bleomycin, busulfan, chlorambucil, cyclophosphamide, melphalan, methotrexate, nitrosureas, procarbazine, vinca alkaloids (with mitomycin), gefitinib, erlotinib
Pleural effusion	Bleomycin, busulfan, interleukin-2, methotrexate, mitomycin, procarbazine
Pulmonary vascular injury	Busulfan, nitrosureas

Adapted with permission from Belknap SM, Kuzel TM, Yarnold PR, et al: Clinical features and correlates of gemcitabine-associated lung injury. Cancer 2006; 106: 2051–2057

Both erlotinib and gefitinib, new oral agents targeted at the epidermal growth factor receptor 1, both have a low (<1%) but real incidence of interstitial pneumonitis that resolves if the agent is stopped. The highest incidence is in Asian patients, where 3.5% of patients may develop interstitial disease also referred to as ground glass opacities, which carries a mortalilty of 1.6%.[13]

HEPATOTOXICITY

The liver is a frequent organ for toxicity with cancer chemotherapeutic agents. Centrilobular hepatocyte injury is the frequent histological finding, elevated transaminases the biochemical manifestation. Antimetabolite drugs such as cytosine arabinoside, methotrexate, hydroxycarbamide and 6-Mercaptopurine are all associated with hepatic injury. 6-Mercaptopurine produces a cholestatic picture, with an elevated alkaline phosphatase and bilirubin. L-Asparaginase and carmustine cause hepatotoxicity as well. The injury reverses with discontinuation of the drug. Chronic methotrexate administration, such as in the treatment of autoimmune diseases, is associated with irreversible fibrosis and cirrhosis.

Hepatic vascular injury is another type of injury to the liver associated with cancer chemotherapeutic agents. Hepatic veno-occlusive disease may occur in up to 20% of patients receiving high-dose chemotherapy in conjunction with bone marrow transplantation, with a mortality up to 50%. Jaundice, ascites and hepatomegaly are the full manifestations of veno-occlusive disease but right upper quadrant pain and weight gain occur more frequently. Obliteration of the central hepatic venules and resulting pressure necrosis of the hepatocytes is seen at autopsy. Many regimens and many individual drugs have been implicated. With busulfan, adjustment of the plasma concentration–time profile may reduce the risk. Dacarbazine, a monofunctional alkylating agent, may produce an eosinophilic centrilobular injury with hepatic vein thromboses.

GASTROINTESTINAL TOXICITY

Chemotherapy-induced diarrhoea has been described with several drugs including the fluoropyrimidines (particularly 5-FU), irinotecan, methotrexate and cisplatin. However, it is the major toxicity of regimens containing a fluoropyrimidine and/or irinotecan that can be dose limiting. Both 5-FU and irinotecan cause acute damage to the intestinal mucosa, leading to loss of epithelium. 5-FU causes a mitotic arrest of crypt cells, leading to an increase in the ratio of immature secretory crypt cells to mature villous enterocytes. The increased volume of fluid that leaves the small bowel exceeds the absorptive capacity of the colon, leading to clinically significant diarrhoea.

In patients treated with irinotecan, early-onset diarrhoea, which occurs during or within several hours of drug infusion in 45–50% of patients, is cholinergically mediated. This effect is thought to be due to structural similarity with acetylcholine. In contrast, late irinotecan-associated diarrhoea is not cholinergically mediated. The pathophysiology of late diarrhoea appears to be multifactorial with contributions from dysmotility and secretory factors as well as a direct toxic effect of the drug on the intestinal mucosa.

Irinotecan produces mucosal changes associated with apoptosis, such as epithelial vacuolization, and goblet cell hyperplasia, suggestive of mucin hypersecretion. These changes appear to be related to the accumulation of the active metabolite of irinotecan, SN-38, in the intestinal mucosa. SN-38 is glucuronidated in the liver and is then excreted in the bile. The conjugated metabolite SN-38G does not appear to cause diarrhoea. However, SN-38G can be deconjugated in the intestines by β-glucuronidase present in intestinal bacteria. A direct correlation has been noted between mucosal damage and either low glucuronidation rates or increased intestinal β-glucuronidase activity. Severe toxicity has been described following irinotecan therapy in patients with Gilbert's syndrome, who have defective hepatic glucuronidation. Experimental studies have shown that inhibition of intestinal β-glucuronidase activity with antibiotics protects against mucosal injury and ameliorates the diarrhoea.

Several recently approved receptor tyrosine kinase inhibitors have diarrhoea associated with use, including sorafenib, sunitinib, erlotinib and gefitinib. The frequency varies from 30–40% with less than 5% grade 3 (severe).[14] Also, rare cases of gastrointestinal perforation have been reported using new agents with several mechanisms of action, including inhibitors of tumour vasculature.[15] Hypertension and rare strokes are also side effects that have been reported.

NEUROTOXICITY

Neurotoxicity from cancer chemotherapeutic agents is an increasingly recognized consequence of cancer treatment. The toxicities observed may affect the brain and spinal cord (CNS), peripheral nerves or the supporting neurological tissues such as the meninges. Neurotoxicity from cancer therapeutic drugs must be distinguished from the effects of space-occupying metastatic lesions, toxic metabolic effects from disorders of blood chemistry, adjunctive drugs (such as opiate narcotics) and paraneoplastic syndromes. Toxicity may be acute, subacute or chronic, reversible or irreversible.

The direct-acting alkylating agents ifosfamide and carmustine cause somnolence, confusion and coma at high doses. The toxicity of ifosfamide is secondary to accumulation of a metabolite, chlorethyl aldehyde, in cerebrospinal fluid. Renal dysfunction may cause CNS toxicity at low doses when acidosis results in increased chlorethyl aldehyde levels.

Damage from the antimetabolite methotrexate occurs in three forms and is worse when given intrathecally with radiation. Chemical arachnoiditis, characterized by headache, fever and nuchal rigidity, is the most common and most acute toxicity. This may be due to additives in the diluent (benzoic acid in sterile water). Subacute toxicity is delayed for 2–3 weeks after administration and is characterized by extremity motor paralysis, cranial nerve palsy seizures and coma. This is due to prolonged exposure to high doses of methotrexate. Chronic demyelinating encephalitis produces dementia and spasticity. There is cortical thinning with enlarged ventricles and cerebral calcifications. Types 2 and 3 may be increased after irradiation especially if concomitant systemic therapy with high (or intermediate) doses is used.

Cytosine arabinoside, when given at high doses, produces cerebral and cerebellar dysfunction due to Purkinje cell necrosis and damage. At standard doses, leukoencephalopathy occurs rarely. When given intrathecally, cytosine arabinoside can produce transverse myelitis with resulting paralysis. 5-FU may produce acute cerebellar toxicity due to inhibition of aconitase, an enzyme in the cerebellar Krebs cycle. The purine adenine deaminase inhibitors pentostatin and fludarabine may produce several types of neurotoxicity. Pentostatin produces somnolence and coma at high doses. Fludarabine may cause delayed-onset coma or cortical blindness at high doses, peripheral neuropathy at low doses. Peripheral neuropathy is a frequent toxicity encountered with many cancer chemotherapeutic agents of many classes. Cisplatin and oxaliplatin, the vinca alkaloids and the taxanes all produce peripheral neuropathy in a cumulative dose-dependent manner (see p.73-76 for more on oxaliplatin-related neurotoxicity).

NEPHROTOXICITY

One of the most serious side-effects of chemotherapeutic agents is nephrotoxicity. Any part of the kidney structure (e.g. the glomerulus, the tubules, the interstitium or the renal microvasculature) could be vulnerable to damage. The clinical manifestations of nephrotoxicity can range from an asymptomatic elevation of serum creatinine to acute renal failure requiring dialysis. Intravascular volume depletion secondary to ascites, oedema or external losses, concomitant use of nephrotoxic drugs, urinary tract obstruction secondary to the underlying malignancy, tumour infiltration of the kidney and intrinsic renal disease can potentiate renal dysfunction in the cancer patient.

Platinum compounds are the agents most associated with renal toxicity. Cisplatin is one of the most commonly used and effective chemotherapeutic agents available and also the best studied antineoplastic nephrotoxic drug. It is a potent tubular toxin, particularly in a low chloride environment, such as the interior of cells. Cell death results via apoptosis or necrosis as DNA-damaged cells enter the cell cycle. Approximately 25–35% of patients will develop a mild and partially reversible decline in renal function after the first course of therapy. The incidence and severity of renal failure increase with subsequent courses, eventually becoming in part irreversible. As a result, discontinuing therapy is generally indicated in those patients who develop a progressive rise in plasma creatinine concentration. In addition to this rise, potentially irreversible hypomagnesaemia due to urinary magnesium wasting may occur in over one-half of cases.

There is suggestive evidence that the nephrotoxicity of cisplatin can be diminished by vigorous hydration and perhaps by giving the drug in a hypertonic solution. A high chloride concentration may minimize both the formation of the highly reactive platinum compounds described above and the uptake of cisplatin by the renal tubular cells. Amifostine, an organic thiophosphate, appears to diminish cisplatin-induced toxicity by donating a protective thiol group, an effect that is highly selective for normal, but not malignant, tissue. Discontinuation of platinum therapy once the plasma creatinine concentration begins to rise should prevent progressive renal failure.

Carboplatin has been synthesized as a non-nephrotoxic platinum analogue, but even though it is less nephrotoxic, it is not free of potential for renal injury. Hypomagnesaemia appears to be the most common manifestation of nephrotoxicity. Other, less common renal side-effects include recurrent salt wasting. No significant clinical nephrotoxicity due to oxaliplatin has yet been reported. Limited data have shown no exacerbation of pre-existing mild renal impairment. Studies of oxaliplatin in patients with progressive degrees of renal failure are in progress.

Cyclophosphamide may produce significant side-effects involving the urinary bladder (haemorrhagic cystitis). The primary renal effect of this agent is hyponatraemia, which is due to impairment of the ability of the kidney to excrete water. The mechanism appears to be due to a direct effect of cyclophosphamide on the distal tubule and not to increased levels of antidiuretic hormone. Hyponatraemia usually occurs acutely and resolves upon discontinuation of the drug (approximately 24 hours). It is recommended that isotonic saline be infused prior to cyclophosphamide administration in order to ameliorate this effect.

Ifosfamide nephrotoxicity has a primary renal effect to produce tubular renal toxicity. The damage produced by ifosfamide is concentrated in the proximal renal tubule and a Fanconi syndrome has been observed after therapy. Other clinical syndromes that have been associated with ifosfamide include nephrogenic diabetes insipidus, renal tubular acidosis and rickets. Pre-existing renal disease is an important risk factor for ifosfamide nephrotoxicity.

Carmustine, lomustine and semustine are lipid-soluble nitrosureas, which have been used against brain tumours. The exact mechanism of nephrotoxicity, however, is incompletely understood. High doses of semustine in children and adults have been associated with progressive renal dysfunction to marked renal insufficiency 3–5 years after therapy. The characteristic histological changes include glomerular sclerosis without immune deposits and interstitial fibrosis. The incidence of nephrotoxicity was reported at 26% in patients with malignant melanoma treated with methyl CCNU in the adjuvant setting. Nephrotoxicity has been reported in 65–75% of patients treated with streptozotocin for prolonged periods of time. Proteinuria is often the first sign of renal damage. This is followed by signs of proximal tubular damage, such as phosphaturia, glycosuria, aminoaciduria, uricosuria and bicarbonaturia. Renal toxicity lasts approximately 2–3 weeks after discontinuing the drug.

The most common form of nephrotoxicity associated with mitomycin C is haemolytic uraemic syndrome. It has been reported in patients who were treated with total doses of mitomycin C in excess of 60 mg/m^2. The renal damage caused by this antineoplastic agent appears to be direct endothelial damage. The incidence of this syndrome ranges from 4% to 6% of patients who receive this drug alone or in combination.

Low or standard doses of methotrexate are usually not associated with renal toxicity, unless patients have underlying renal dysfunction. High doses (1–15 g/m^2) are associated with a 47% incidence of renal toxicity, accompanied by methotrexate crystals in the urine. The mechanism for methotrexate-induced nephrotoxicity is explained in part by its limited solubility at an acid pH, which leads to intratubular precipitation. Patients who are volume depleted and excrete an acidic urine are at higher risk for nephrotoxicity. With aggressive hydration and urine alkalinization, the incidence of renal failure with high doses of methotrexate can be decreased. The clinical picture of methotrexate-induced renal failure is that of a non-oliguric renal failure. Preventive measures when using high doses of methotrexate include aggressive intravenous hydration with saline and urine alkalinization with sodium bicarbonate to maintain a urine pH around 7.0. If renal failure develops, methotrexate levels will increase and the risk of systemic toxicity will also be enhanced. In addition to supportive measures, patients should be started on folinic acid rescue, until levels of methotrexate fall below 0.5 uM.

VEGF or VEGFR2-targeted agents produce albuminuria in 10–25% of patients, sometimes to nephrotic range. The exact mechanism has not been elucidated but studies in mice with conditional expression of VEGF in the podocytes confirms a major role for VEGF in endothelial development and maintainence of a fenestrated endothelium.[16] Like hypertension, this appears to be a class effect but the factors associated with occurrence and severity are unknown. If clinically significant, decreasing the dose or discontinuation of drug are the only current approaches.

LATE COMPLICATIONS OF CANCER CHEMOTHERAPY

As cancer therapy has become increasingly effective and more patients live longer, late complications have become apparent separate from the direct toxic effects on organ system function described above. Gonadal dysfunction is one. In males, the primary lesion is depletion of germinal epithelium of seminiferous tubules with marked decrease in testicular volume, oligo- or azoospermia and infertility. There is an increase in follicle-stimulating hormone (FSH) and occasionally in luteinizing hormone (LH). No change is seen in serum testosterone. Alkylating agents (and irradiation) are the most damaging and toxicity is dose related. About 80% of males with Hodgkin's disease treated with MOPP are oligo-azoospermic. About half recover in up to 4 years. Procarbazine is a major offender. Anthracyclines also cause azoospermia in a dose-related fashion. In females, the primary lesion is ovarian fibrosis and follicle destruction. Amenorrhoea ensues, with increase in FSH and LH and a decrease in oestradiol leading to vaginal atrophy and endometrial hypoplasia. Onset and duration are dose and age related. Alkylating agents (and irradiation) again are the worst offenders.

In children, the prepubertal effects may be less profound and reversible in males, though the pubertal effects may be more severe with often irreversible azoospermia, decreased testosterone and increased FSH and LH. Less is known about females, but young girls appear quite resistant to alkylating agents.

No more tragic toxicity is seen with cancer chemotherapeutic agents than the induction of a second, treatment-related cancer in a patient cured of one cancer.[17,18] Of the wide variety of environmental and chemical agents causing cancer, there is one common thread in their mode of action – interaction with DNA. Clinical studies detailing this consequence of therapy have many problems, including the inherent bias of reporting index cases, the retrospective nature of many reports, the lack of reliable information on drug dosage, total amount of drug given and duration of therapy and the underlying incidence of second malignancy. The direct-acting alkylating agents are most often implicated and chronic, low-dose administration is a greater risk factor. Acute non-lymphocytic leukaemia or myelodysplasia is the best described. The indirect-acting topoisomerase II agents produce a specific 11q23 translocation.

Osteonecrosis of the jaw has been seen with increasing frequency during the past few years, related in part to chronic use of intravenous bisphophonates for advanced cancer. The incidence has been estimated at 1–10% of patients receiving these medications.[19] The pathogenesis and optimal management for osteonecrosis of the jaw are poorly understood, with multiple risk factors and various treatments involved.[20]

REFERENCES

1. Weiss RB: Toxicity of chemotherapy – the last decade. Semin Oncol 2006; 33: 1.
2. Crawford J, Cella D, Sonis ST: Managing chemotherapy-related side effects: trends in the use of cytokines and other growth factors. Oncology 2006; 20: Suppl.
3. Zorzou MP, Efstathiou E, Galani E, et al: Carboplatin hypersensitivity reactions. J Chemother 2005; 17(1): 104–110.
4. Cristaaudo A, Sera F, Severino V, et al: Occupational hypersensitivity to metal salts, including platinum, in the secondary industry. Allergy 2005; 60(2): 138–139.
5. Szebeni J: Complement activation-related pseudoallergy: a new class of drug induced acute immune toxicity. Toxicology 2005; 216: 106–121.
6. Escudier B, Szczylik C, Eisen T, et al: Randomized phase III trial of the Raf kinase and VEGFR inhibitor sorafenib (BAY 43-9006) in patients with advanced renal cell carcinoma (RCC). J Clin Oncol 2005; 23(18 Suppl): abstract 4510.
7. Perez-Solar R, Saltz L. Cutaneous adverse effects with HER1/EGFR-targeted agents: is there a silver lining? J Clin Oncol 2005; 23(24): 5235–5246.
8. Floyd JD, Nguyen DT, Lobins RL, et al: Cardiotoxicity of cancer therapy. J Clin Oncol 2005; 23: 7685–7696.

9. Kerkela R, Grazette L, Yacobi R, et al: Cardiotoxicity of the cancer therapeutic agent imatinib mesylate. Nat Med 2006; 12(8): 908–916.

10. Hurwitz H: Integrating the anti-VEGF – A humanized monoclonal antibody bevacizumab with chemotherapy in advanced colorectal cancer. Clin Colorectal Cancer 2004; 4 Suppl 2: S62–S68.

11. Motzer RJ, Hutson TE, Tomczak P, et al: Phase III randomized trial of sunitinib malate (SU11248) versus interferon alfa as first line systemic therapy for patients with metastatic renal cell carcinoma. J Clin Oncol 2006; 24 (18 Suppl): 930s abstract LBA3.

12. Belknap SM, Kuzel TM, Yarnold PR, et al: Clinical features and correlates of gemcitabine-associated lung injury. Cancer 2006; 106: 2051–2057.

13. Ando M, Okamoto I, Yamamoto N, et al: Predictive factors for interstitial lung disease, antitumor response, and survival in non-small-cell lung cancer patients treated with gefitinib. J Clin Oncol 2006; 24: 2549–2556.

14. Niho S, Kubota K, Goto K, et al: First-line single agent treatment with gefitinib in patients with advanced non-small cell lung cancer: a phase II study. J Clin Oncol 2006; 24(1): 64–69.

15. Ratain MJ, Eisen T, Stadler WM, et al: Phase II placebo-controlled randomized discontinuation trial of sorafenib in patients with metastatic renal cell carcinoma. J Clin Oncol 2006; 24: 2505–2512.

16. Erimina V, Quaggin SE: The role of VEGF-A in glomerular development and function. Curr Opin Nephrol Hypertens 2004; 13: 9–15.

17. Bhatia S, Landier W: Evaluating survivors of pediatric cancer. Cancer J 2005; 11: 340–354.

18. Hudson MM, Mertens AC, Yasui Y, et al: Health status in adults treated for childhood cancer: a report from the childhood survivor study. Am J Oncol Rev 2004; 3: 165–170.

19. Badros A, Weikel D, Salama A, et al: Osteonecrosis of the jaw in multiple myeloma patients: clinical features and risk factors. J Clin Oncol 2006; 24: 945–952.

20. Ruggiero S, Gralow J, Marx RE, et al. Practical guidelines for the prevention, diagnosis and treatment of osteonecrosis of the jaw in patients with cancer. J Oncol Pract 2006; 2: 7–14.

FURTHER READING

Adrian RM, Hood, AF, Skarin AT. Mucocutaneous reactions to antineoplastic agents. CA Cancer J Clin 1980; 30: 143–157.

Attar EC, Ervin T, Janicek M, Deykin A, Godleski J: Acute interstitial pneumonitis related to gemcitabine. J Clin Oncol 2000; 18: 697–698.

Burstein H: Radiation recall dermatitis from gemcitabine. J Clin Oncol 2000; 18: 693–694.

Chabner BA, Longo DL: Cancer Chemotherapy and Biotherapy, 2nd edn. Lippincott–Raven, Philadelphia, 1996.

Darnell J, Lodish H, Baltimore D: Molecular Cell Biology, 3rd edn. W.H. Freeman, New York, 1995.

DeVita VT, Jr, Hellman S, Rosenberg SA: Cancer: Principles and Practice of Oncology, 4th edn. Lippincott, Philadelphia, 1993.

Eder JP: Neoplasms. In: Page CP, Curtis MJ, Sutter MC, Walker MJA, Hoffman BB, eds: Integrated Pharmacology. Mosby–Times Mirror International, London, 1997: 501–522.

Hussain S, Anderson DN, Salvatti ME, et al: Onycholysis as a complication of systemic chemotherapy. Cancer 2000; 88: 2367–2371.

Perry MD: The Chemotherapy Source Book. Williams and Wilkins, Baltimore, 1992.

Skeel RT: Handbook of Cancer Chemotherapy. Little, Brown, Boston, 1991.

Sonis ST, Fey EG: Oral complications of cancer therapy. Oncology 2002; 16: 680–691.

Index